W9-ABI-354

Arnold Melnick, DO

Professionally Speaking
Public Speaking
for Health Professionals

Pre-publication
REVIEWS,
COMMENTARIES,
EVALUATIONS . . .

"**A**lthough I have been professionally speaking for over forty years, I have never consciously thought about all the things one has to do in order to make a first-rate medical presentation. Dr. Melnick's book has managed to touch on virtually everything one needs to think about when preparing to communicate medical issues to an audience. I wish that it was available years ago. It certainly would have helped me be an even better medical speaker."

Bernard J. Fogel, MD
Senior Advisor to the President
and Dean Emeritus,
University of Miami School of Medicine

"**A**n easy reading, very practical 'how to—what not to' approach to public speaking for health care professionals. Dr. Melnick has clearly given many public addresses, some under rather 'trying conditions.' His appreciation for detail, enjoyable sense of humor, and genuine enthusiasm for effectively communicating are evident. Health care professionals have much to contribute to society. How to accomplish this laudable objective is the challenge. The practical tips provided will be useful for novices and experienced presenters. The uninformed may consider public speaking a 'gift' or an 'art,' yet there is considerable groundwork that must first be done to achieve success. Communicating with the public is clearly an important aspect of professionalism, but one that, unfortunately, is almost never addressed during training."

Pat DeLeon
Past Recording Secretary,
American Psychological Association

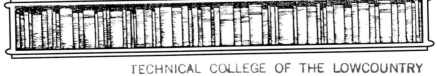

TECHNICAL COLLEGE OF THE LOWCOUNTRY
LEARNING RESOURCES CENTER
POST OFFICE BOX 1288
BEAUFORT, SOUTH CAROLINA 29901-1288

NOTES FOR PROFESSIONAL LIBRARIANS AND LIBRARY USERS

This is an original book title published by The Haworth Press, Inc. Unless otherwise noted in specific chapters with attribution, materials in this book have not been previously published elsewhere in any format or language.

CONSERVATION AND PRESERVATION NOTES

All books published by The Haworth Press, Inc. and its imprints are printed on certified pH neutral, acid free book grade paper. This paper meets the minimum requirements of American National Standard for Information Sciences–Permanence of Paper for Printed Material, ANSI Z39.48-1984.

Professionally Speaking
Public Speaking
for Health Professionals

THE HAWORTH PRESS

Advances in Psychology and Mental Health
Frank De Piano, PhD
Senior Editor

Beyond the Therapeutic Relationship: Behavioral, Biological, and Cognitive Foundations of Psychotherapy by Frederic J. Leger

How the Brain Talks to Itself: A Clinical Primer of Psychotherapeutic Neuroscience by Jay E. Harris

Cross-Cultural Counseling: The Arab-Palestinian Case by Marwan Dwairy

The Vulnerable Therapist: Practicing Psychotherapy in an Age of Anxiety by Helen W. Coale

Professionally Speaking: Public Speaking for Health Professionals by Arnold Melnick

Introduction to Group Therapy: A Practical Guide by Scott Simon Fehr

Professionally Speaking
Public Speaking
for Health Professionals

Arnold Melnick, DO

The Haworth Press
New York • London

TECHNICAL COLLEGE OF THE LOWCOUNTRY
LEARNING RESOURCES CENTER
POST OFFICE BOX 1288
BEAUFORT, SOUTH CAROLINA 29901-1288

© 1998 by The Haworth Press, Inc. All rights reserved. No part of this work may be reproduced or utilized in any form or by any means, electronic or mechanical, including photocopying, microfilm, and recording, or by any information storage and retrieval system, without permission in writing from the publisher. Printed in the United States of America.

The Haworth Press, Inc., 10 Alice Street, Binghamton, NY 13904-1580

Cover design by Jennifer M. Gaska.

Library of Congress Cataloging-in-Publication Data

Melnick, Arnold.
    Professionally speaking : public speaking for health professionals / Arnold Melnick.
        p.   cm.
    Includes index.
    ISBN 0-7890-0601-4 (alk. paper).
    1. Public speaking. 2. Medical personnel. I. Title.
PN4192.M43M45 1998
808.5′1′02461—dc21

98-22026
CIP

I dedicate this book to my late father, David Melnick, a speaker *par excellence,* without any formal training whatsoever—and a role model for me; to my wife, Anita, ever my severest and most constructive critic and ardent supporter; and to my family, Sandy, Nona, Rachel, and Steven, who make it all worthwhile.

ABOUT THE AUTHOR

Arnold Melnick, DO, MSc, DHL (Honorary), recently retired as Executive Vice Chancellor and Provost, Health Professions Division, at Nova Southeastern University in Ft. Lauderdale, Florida. Throughout two careers—in Pediatrics and Medical Education—Dr. Melnick's activities led him into many aspects of professional public speaking, including teaching at medical school and hospital levels. He has earned five fellowship degrees, served as president or chairman of ten regional or national professional groups, and received ten distinguished service awards. He has taught in three medical schools and has served as Professor of Pediatrics, of Public Health, and of Medical Communications. He has been involved in many important governmental and academic committees and organizations dealing with medical and education issues. Known for his lucid, lively, and often humorous presentations—whether medical or otherwise—he has lectured extensively in almost every state in America, at a number of institutions, and for many organizations, including several honors lectures. His topics have included medical subjects, socioeconomics related to medicine and "lay" lectures, and he has served as presiding officer or master of ceremonies on innumerable occasions and as host for over 700 instructional tapes. Dr. Melnick is also a writer with more than sixty articles and a published book on pediatrics to his credit. He is a past president of the American Medical Writers Association (AMWA) and its Mid-Atlantic chapter.

CONTENTS

Foreword

Arnold Melnick and I go back a long time in the practice of medicine in Philadelphia. When I was a young pediatric surgeon, not only trying to make his mark, but to justify the specialty of pediatric surgery, Arnold Melnick was an enthusiastic referring physician. This was in the days when the relationship between osteopathic physicians and allopathic physicians was not as cordial as it is today, but that was not the case with Drs. Melnick and Koop.

I spoke for Arnold Melnick on the specialty of pediatric surgery at osteopathic meetings, he supported me by referring patients for surgery, and I in turn, as he advanced academically, began to train osteopathic surgeons in pediatric surgery at the Children's Hospital of Philadelphia.

Although the pursuit of our own academic careers has led us further and further apart geographically, we have never lost contact, nor have we lost our shared concern that all professionals could be better communicators with very little effort along practical lines. Arnold Melnick has pursued this concern and has produced a readable series of hints and suggestions to make the professional health speaker a more articulate communicator. The result is *Professionally Speaking: Public Speaking for Health Professionals.*

It is especially appropriate that Dr. Melnick's book arrives on the scene at this time when the information explosion is making it possible for more and more patients to be taught how to take charge of their health. And in today's area this transition in health care will take some effort and it will take commitment from the health professions to do a better job of communicating, not only with fellow professionals, but with the public as well.

That is what this book is all about. I am sure it will help any who use it. Dr. Melnick has contributed a great service to us who either speak professionally or wish we could do it better.

At the very least no one that reads this book can say, "I do not know how!"

C. Everett Koop, MD, ScD

Preface

All of us speak continually. We speak to our friends and colleagues. We speak to our families and to strangers. We speak formally and informally. Most of the time we do all of this so easily and unconsciously, without any major difficulties, that we consider it natural. We generally feel no need for training or assistance.

However, when it comes to medical or professional speaking (or other forms of public speaking), we sometimes encounter difficulties. Someone once said, "Man is an animal whose brain starts to work before birth and doesn't stop until he stands up to speak." For this kind of speaking, many people do need some help. That is the purpose of this book.

What do I mean by "professionally speaking"? Medical or professional speaking is any kind of presentation or discussion on medical or other professional subjects from any sort of "platform" in front of an audience. It may be a lecture, a symposium, or a panel discussion; it may be a classroom presentation. The audience may be small or large. Regardless, it is professional speaking.

In this context, individual differences in ability become so much more evident. In trying to rationalize these differences, we often make assumptions about what creates them, generally based on prejudices or myths. Is it talent? Or is it training? This is the old debate of heredity versus environment, a basic issue in so many things. Are good speakers born good speakers? Does environment make good speakers out of those with less talent? Can you become a good speaker through training?

I have specific feelings about these questions. I believe strongly that some people have so much innate talent that they are excellent speakers without any kind of training and regardless of whether or not they observe what might be called "the rules." They are generally the "stars." Most of us have some latent natural ability that can be considerably improved by concentration, motivation, practice, help, or training. (As an analogy, remember that people can be in excellent health through a fortunate genetic inheritance that predisposes them to good health; however, even this good health can be improved by "assistance" and "training," that is, medical advice and help.)

This book is written to aid those people who want help in improving their professional speaking. Remember that truly natural speakers may do things completely different from the suggestions incorporated in this book. That is okay. For beginners, however, or for speakers who wish to improve themselves, I offer this book.

Most of all, this book is written for those who are at least somewhat serious about improving their ability. To those without that motivation, many of the ideas may seem too intense or too difficult. For those who are motivated for improvement, I hope my approach will help.

Most of the suggestions contained in this book arise from whatever basic ability I may have inherited, enhanced by the many outstanding role models I have observed, plus my own personal experiences over many years.

I have tried to integrate all the sources in my background into an understandable approach to *Professionally Speaking.* Some of the material in this book comes from long-forgotten sources, read or heard, which have become so much a part of me that I cannot recall where or when I learned them. To those anonymous contributors to my life, I am most grateful.

I also must acknowledge the dedicated and valuable contribution of my former Executive Assistant, Susan Darcy Peake, for typing and retyping and for so much other work on this book.

Chapter 1

Types of Professional Talks

THE FOUR TYPES OF TALKS

Memorized Talk

This type of talk is rarely used, especially in a substantial presentation. It requires too much time; it is fraught with great danger because the failure to remember leads to unneeded embarrassment; it usually becomes an inferior form of presentation, unless the speaker is a trained actor.

However, it must be pointed out that there may be instances in which a speaker will want to memorize a certain passage (a poem, a quotation) or certain statistics to be used in the talk. The memorized talk is so poor a possibility for medical speaking that no further mention of it will be made in this book.

Manuscript Talk

This is a talk in which the speaker reads verbatim from a written manuscript. The speaker might have prepared a written paper (for publication) and, when asked to present it orally, decided to read the paper to the group. Or, the speaker may prepare a speech especially written for the occasion and then read it to the audience. The speaker may commission an outsider (especially one skilled in writing speeches) to prepare a manuscript for this presentation. The first two are very frequent occurrences at professional meetings, and the last is rather rare. Because of the frequency of the first two, more will be described about them later in the book.

Extemporaneous Talk

Some dictionaries define *extemporaneous* as carefully prepared but delivered without notes or text. They also offer *impromptu* as a synonym. Certainly, there is a great deal of semantics in defining these two words and differentiating them.

For purposes of clarity in this book, I shall use relatively common meanings. *Extemporaneous* will be used to mean prepared (either with or without notes or text) but delivered without writing out the specific words.

Here, too, there are a number of variations. Some speakers may prepare a fully written manuscript for the talk and then use it as an outline or prompter for the extemporaneous talk. Very often, when this is done, the speaker may "mark up" his manuscript to serve as a sort of outline during the speech. Other speakers may prepare outlines (of varying kinds) to serve as prompters for their talk.

Impromptu Talk

Impromptu here will be used here to mean an on-the-spot, improvised presentation where there is no formal preparation—only an accumulation of knowledge that permits the speaker to call on this background on the spur of the moment.

All these talks require preparation in varying degrees and varying amounts. In those written out or outlined, the preparation is obvious. The impromptu talk requires some background and a pool of knowledge from which to draw, either as a spur-of-the-moment commentary or in reply to questions. For example, I could never give an impromptu talk on architecture, or carpentry, or nuclear science. I have no background, and therefore, an impromptu talk is impossible. However, in the field of medicine, at least some certain aspects of medicine, I could answer questions or make a spontaneous commentary if called upon to do so.

Probably the most famous story about impromptu talks concerned Daniel Webster, one of the greatest orators who ever served in the U.S. Senate. On one particular day, a subject came up about which Daniel Webster felt strongly. He rose to his feet, asked for the floor, and gave one of his brilliant orations; it lasted almost three hours. When he finished, he was surrounded by well-wishers, one of whom asked, "Senator Webster, how long did it take you to write that speech?" Webster looked at the questioner briefly and replied, "Thirty years, thirty years."

My readers may question where teaching in professional school fits into this classification. Although most of this book is devoted to other kinds of presentations, the professional lecture is usually an extemporaneous presentation, with instructors using outlines or audiovisual slides to focus on a prepared subject. For the most part, reading of a manuscript occurs rarely, and when it does, the result is almost disastrous. Impromptu talks, even by an instructor who has a fabulous background in the subject, generally show lack of concern for the audience; they will almost never be adequately organized and should never be used.

Chapter 2

Writing a Professional Speech

The aim of a professional speech is to create the best communication between the speaker and the audience. Oral and written communication are different so writing a medical paper for oral presentation requires skills in addition to the usual writing skills. In many instances, this means modifying a published paper so that the listeners' absorption and understanding is maximum.

Why is an oral presentation different? It is obvious that the listeners cannot go back and reread a sentence or word they have missed. They must be able to have instantaneous recognition and understanding of the words and thoughts as they are being spoken. In order to achieve this, the writing must be different from the usual published presentation. In fact, the manuscript should always reflect the speaking style of the speaker, whether he or she is doing the writing or not.

Does this mean that a splendidly written (published or about-to-be published) paper cannot be read? First, most of us have an exaggerated idea of how "splendidly written" our articles are once they have been accepted for publication. Second, most papers written for publication are deliberately made to be understandable to the eye (and not to the ear, which is different). Third, because of the first two reasons, the words and phrases themselves tend to be flat and boring and require the investment of much concentration and energy for a listener to comprehend. And fourth, these three may sometimes combine with what may be a dull, uninteresting reading style that puts the audience to sleep.

Thus, I recommend that a speech written for publication never be read to an audience. Further, if a professional talk is to be read, either prepare it de novo or rewrite the publication paper to put it in proper condition for reading.

WRITING THE TALK

First, I highly recommend that speeches being prepared for delivery should originally be tape recorded using a dictating machine. We human beings can think at least five times as fast as we can handwrite, and we have a tendency in writing to edit as we go along. This creates two problems. First, the editing interferes with the smooth flow of thought that the writer has initially. By the time you write down your thoughts, and do even light editing as you write, you often forget what you had in mind. Second, the slower pace of writing (or typing) slows down the entire process. Dictating is preferred also because this type of composition will reflect your style of speech. However, I must emphasize that very few people can turn out a finished speech manuscript with a single dictation, anymore than most people can turn out a finished manuscript for publication in one writing. Therefore, the manuscript for a speech must be rewritten (no matter which method you use for the first draft), perhaps several times. It needs rewriting for accuracy of thought and word, and it needs rewriting to be certain it is understandable to the ear.

Since listeners have a shorter attention span than readers and cannot refer back to words or thoughts already spoken, the manuscript must be carefully reviewed from the standpoint of the listener.

What then are some of the clues to making a manuscript better for speech than for publication?

- A manuscript for speech should contain shorter sentences, and they must have absolute clarity.
- The manuscript should contain both simple and compound sentences. Complex sentences may be used from time to

time for variety, but the author must be absolutely sure that they are clear and have no confusing parts to them. Use fewer of them than in a manuscript for publication. (This paragraph is a good example of the mix of sentences.)

- A manuscript for speech should contain stronger, punchier words.
- Watch out for "whiches." These generally prolong sentences and confuse the listener. It is much better to make separate sentences because the listener may have difficulty identifying the antecedent of the "which." Try reading to someone the following sentence: "The patient vomited and I gave him medication which caused him to be very thirsty." Just in reading this, confusion abounds. How much more complicated it is to decipher this statement purely by listening.
- Watch out for "this" or "that" when they are used to refer to a complex antecedent. They present the same problem as "which." Think about listening to this sentence: "I gave the patient penicillin and a venoclysis as treatment for infection. This complicated his hospital stay." What does "this" refer to? Penicillin? Venoclysis? Infection? If it's ambiguous when reading it, think about how it sounds.
- For similar reasons, a speaker should never make references using words such as "former," "latter," "above," "previous," or similar words. Again, in reading, you can look back to see what the word refers to. But in listening, there is no looking back. These references are to previously spoken ideas, and the listener may already have lost track of them. It is far better to repeat, in a capsule word or phrase, the idea that you are referring to so that there is no question in the listener's mind which idea you mean. You can say, "that program" instead of "the former" or "my therapeutic approach" rather than "the latter."
- The same care applies to personal pronouns.

- Avoid stumble words. These are words with which a particular speaker may have difficulty because of the combination of vowels and consonants that occur. Not everyone has the same difficulties in speaking, and you will have to identify those words or phrases you are likely to stumble on. There are people who can say, "Peter Piper picked a peck of pickled peppers," without making a single mistake and say it as fast as necessary. On the other hand, there are people who stumble over simple combinations of words such as "especially susceptible," which is one of my stumble phrases. This is an example of why it is necessary to know yourself and your speaking abilities.

- Avoid sibilants. Even the best of speakers gets into difficulty with the "S" sounds, particularly if they occur in series; it may sound like the speaker is whistling. This is made even worse if he or she is using a microphone. Words such as "lawlessness" or "uselessness" should be eliminated if you have the least bit of difficulty with them. "Especially susceptible," referred to previously, is another "whistler." Other phrases should be substituted for them. Learn to know your own speech patterns well.

- Transition words should be used; they greatly help the listeners' understanding. Introductory words such as "now," "however," and others should be used to tie one thought into another for clarity to the listener.

- Simplify all difficult words and symbols. This means substituting simple words for complex words when they mean the same thing, such as "breathe" for "respire." (This is just as applicable in writing for publication.) It also means sometimes using a nonverbal symbol or gesture to help the listener understand. For example, if you are discussing a complex chemical formula, you don't want to repeat the entire formula symbol by symbol each time you say it or use a complex chemical term. If there is not a key word that will describe it, then perhaps writing the formula on a blackboard or projecting it on a screen and pointing to it each time will make it clear. Or, you might refer to it each time by such a term as "this compound."

- In writing for listening, you should only use the first and second person (I, me, you) and never impersonal words such as "one," "this researcher," or "this writer." These are stilted and confusing. Always use the active voice: this is the way we talk in our normal conversations, and this is the way you should talk from the platform.
- Although references to other publications are frequent in published articles, they appear to be wasted in most talks, unless the publication or writer is of universal stature and known by everybody. Quoting names that are unknown or unrecognizable to most of your audience will not impress them, but it might make them think you are a name-dropper. Allusions to unknown persons or to unknown events or to information known only to the speaker and a specific group will lose the audience and have no value whatsoever. On the other hand, referring to or quoting a universally known authority will be understood and may give authority to your talk.

ALWAYS REMEMBER, YOU ARE TALKING TO A LISTENER!

WRITING FOR OTHERS

To write a speech for someone else, you must know the speaker, for the speech must reflect the personality of the speaker, not the writer. The writer should know the speaker's likes and dislikes, capabilities and limitations. What kinds of humor is the speaker capable of? In what kinds of humor is he or she somewhat restricted? How intellectual is he or she? How populist? The better the writer knows the speaker, the better the speech will be. It is important that the speech reflect the tone and intellect and interests of the speaker in order to be consistent and credible. Good publication writers are not necessarily good speech writers, although they may be.

It should go without saying that the writer is not doing a presentation of his or her own but rather should write the talk as though the speaker had written it. If a speechwriter produces a manuscript that sounds like the speaker's own words, it is a good, well-prepared talk.

Once the manuscript is prepared, the writer must review it with the speaker, and no matter how much "pride of authorship" there is, the writer should never push anything on the speaker if the speaker is uncomfortable with it. It may be necessary (and wise) to review the talk with the speaker several times. It is of equally great value for the speaker to rehearse the talk in front of the writer. This allows for two important things: rehearsal gives both of them an opportunity to check the speech and the presentation, and the writer gains an opportunity to check on the speaker's delivery and to help with the presentation or to do any necessary rewriting.

Finally, having properly prepared the speech, arrangement should be made for the speech to be taped at the time of actual presentation. This tape should be reviewed by the speaker and the writer together, as a sort of postmortem to detect any errors either in writing or delivery that they may have made. This allows them to collaborate for better talks in the future.

Chapter 3

Preparing the Manuscript

One of the aids available to improve the reading of a speech is the mechanical preparation of the manuscript. Proper markings, clues, and reminders to help the speaker will help make the reading of a paper more understandable.

There are many mechanical ways of preparing a manuscript, and whatever suggestions are offered here are not necessarily the best, nor are they etched in stone. The well-motivated speaker can easily come up with novel ideas about preparing the manuscript. Some of the suggestions presented here may even seem too elemental to the reader, and you may ask whether it is necessary to go through all of this "junk" just to give a paper. (If you are going to give a paper, it is worth giving properly.) But the answer to the question is twofold. First, the more experienced the speaker, the less likely he or she will need this kind of mechanical support. Second, marking up a paper for reading is just as important as (and is comparable to) editing a paper for publication.

Television anchorpersons do not need to mark their scripts to tell them where emphasis goes or how to handle certain aspects of their presentations. They have learned to do it very naturally after a great deal of practice, and they are fine examples of reading manuscripts at its best. On the other hand, inexperienced speakers can profit by using as many of these aids as necessary until they learn to do most of it by eye and brain, similar to the television anchors.

Furthermore, it is just as important to use these aids for the reading of a paper as it is to edit and rewrite a manuscript that is being prepared for publication. No one ever achieves perfection, but all serious speakers and writers strive toward it. That means using every available device to reach your goal. If the speech is at all worth giving, worth spending time to deliver, and worth people's coming to hear, then it is worth doing properly; this means spending sufficient time on it, even though the amount of time may be considerable. Unfortunately, in the real world, far less time is spent in preparing speeches than is spent on preparing papers for publication. Perhaps this is because speeches, whether written and read or given spontaneously, are not preserved for posterity. More likely, it is because there is no editor with a blue pencil listening somewhere on the microphone to edit what the speaker is saying and to make sure that the speech comes out properly. As a result of this, most speakers tend to become far more indifferent or casual about preparation to the detriment of their talks.

Some of the human aspects of reading a speech are difficult (nervousness, concentration on subject matter, outside distractions) so speakers are well advised to make use of the mechanical markings to the manuscript to make themselves as comfortable as possible. This greatly reduces the likelihood of error.

Some specific recommendations can be made:

- Whenever possible, the manuscript should be typed with a large typeface and the material should be double-spaced or even triple-spaced. Orator type was invented by IBM for just this purpose, as was Presenter. The letters are considerably larger than any other common typewriter faces and easier to read. If you have any difficulty whatsoever seeing the manuscript page or your vision starts to become less acute as you age (as I can assure you it does), then you will want the largest type possible. This prevents you from making mistakes because you cannot see clearly and, more important, prevents the necessity for you to bend over the podium every time you look at the manuscript, straining to see it.

There are two problems with Orator type: it is too condensed, that is, the letters are spaced too close to one another horizontally, and it is composed of large capital letters and small capital letters rather than capital and lowercase letters (which would be much easier to read) (see Figure 3.1).

For some people, even the use of Orator type (or something similar) will not be quite large enough to make the type clearly visible when standing at the podium. Figure 3.2 shows a mechanism to improve this. First, draw a template (an area guide) approximately four inches wide and six inches high in the center of a sheet of ordinary typing paper. Type the manuscript in Orator type within these bounds (see Figure 3.3). Photocopy this page on an enlarging copy machine, blowing it up to approximately double the size. This will give you a readable manuscript (see Figure 3.4).

- New computer software has aided greatly in the preparation of manuscripts for reading. With it, you can choose type font and size—and printing—with one primary process. Since you, the speaker, are the one who needs to be comfortable with the finished manuscript, so that you can be at ease reading at the podium, it becomes very much a personal choice. At this point, I have found myself most comfortable with computer-set Times Roman at eighteen-point or twenty-point size, and I have used it repeatedly with total satisfaction. Try your own variations and choose what accommodates you best.
- If you are not enlarging Orator type, the individual typed lines should be no longer than approximately six inches, about as much as the human eye can take in at one glance. This avoids excessive eye movement and allows for fast recognition of an entire thought on a single line.
- You should leave a margin of approximately 1½ to 1 inches on the left-hand side of the manuscript. In this space, you can write notes to yourself for the delivery of the paper. Although many speakers will make their delivery notes right

on the manuscript, both above and around the lines, for the beginning speaker it is probably easier to use the space in the left-hand margin for doing this. This margin also provides a place to enter last-minute comments or thoughts.

- All pages should be numbered clearly, preferably in the upper right-hand corner, to identify the continuity of pages without confusion. This also eliminates trying to find the page number if it is at the bottom of the page.
- Pages should never be stapled together; use a paper clip instead. As soon as you put your manuscript on the rostrum, remove the paper clip. When pages are stapled, it becomes necessary to fold the paper each time you turn a page. This creates a clumsy package and makes turning pages more difficult.
- The type of paper used for the manuscript is also important. It should be paper that is sturdy enough not to crinkle in your hands (for example, onionskin paper is a no-no) but not too stiff so that it crinkles if held near a very sensitive microphone.
- Moving from page to page as you talk can also be done in a systematic way. Slide each page to one side as you finish with it so that you are facing two sheets, the one you are presently reading from and the one you have just finished. The finished pile should be to the side and the current pile with the remainder of your speech should be directly in front of you. This allows a smooth transition from the bottom of one page to the top of the next without a lot of shuffling of papers.
- In typing the manuscript, words should not be hyphenated at the end of a line. Word breaks from one line to the other make words more difficult to see and recognize. It is better to end a line with leftover space than to split a word.
- No sentence breaks should occur from one page to the other. This will provide the same ease of reading. Similarly, no paragraph should carry over from one page to the next. Both

paragraphs and sentences should end at the bottom of a page, even if it is necessary to have a lot of empty space at the bottom. This allows you to end thoughts on a page rather than carry them over to the next page and avoids confusing the speaker.

- The end of the speech should be indicated by writing "END" on the manuscript. Sometimes the context of the speech may not suggest that the prepared speech is ending, even though it should if written properly, and often the tension of delivering the speech can cause the speaker to forget.

There are some other devices that have been found helpful. Some speakers prefer to have their manuscripts typed, with each sentence written as a separate paragraph and with lines drawn across the page to indicate the end of each paragraph. This is more often used in political speeches than in scientific speeches. However, this device might help the beginning speaker who needs some assistance. Others have been known to use the mechanism of finishing a page with a large margin at the bottom, with the first four or five words of the following page in the bottom right-hand corner. This, too, helps the speaker in the transition from one page to another.

I repeat my advice that some inexperienced speakers will find it helpful to write instructions for themselves in the left-hand margin. These may include instructions for gestures, mood (such as smiling, seriousness), or any other information that the speaker wants to be certain to remember.

I have included additional recommendations in Chapter 7 for enhancing your manuscript that suggest the utilization of manuscript markings to aid the speaker in remembering important points for delivery.

TECHNICAL COLLEGE OF THE LOWCOUNTRY
LEARNING RESOURCES CENTER
POST OFFICE BOX 1288
BEAUFORT, SOUTH CAROLINA 29901-1288

FIGURE 3.1. Orator and Presenter Typefaces

THIS IS ORATOR TYPEFACE, MANUFACTURED BY IBM.
PLEASE NOTE HOW CLOSE TOGETHER THE LETTERS ARE, BUT
IT IS LARGER THAN MOST TYPEWRITER FONTS.

This is Presenter typeface, made larger by IBM in order to be visible from a greater distance.

FIGURE 3.2. Template for Use in Enlarging Type

FIGURE 3.3. Copy Typed Within Template Bounds

CONTAINING A NUMBER OF COMMON CHARACTERISTICS—UNDERDEVELOPMENT, POVERTY, AND ECONOMIC DEPENDENCE OF THE FIRST TWO WORLDS.

ORIGINALLY SMALL, THE THIRD WORLD COUNTRIES HAVE NOW GROWN TO BE MORE THAN HALF OF THE WORLD'S POPULATION. BY THE BEGINNING OF THE NEXT CENTURY THEY WILL COMPOSE 80 PERCENT OF THE WORLD'S POPULATION.

I PROPOSE THAT THERE IS ALSO A THIRD WORLD IN MEDICINE, TOTALLY ANALOGOUS TO THE POLITICAL UNIVERSE. IT HAS SIMILAR CHARACTERISTICS. IT IS ESSENTIALLY "NOTHING AND WANTS TO BE SOMETHING" AND IT GENERALLY IS ASSOCIATED WITH UNDERDEVELOPMENT, POVERTY, AND

FIGURE 3.4. Enlargement of Template-Size Copy (Double Size)—
Readability Is Now Greater

CONTAINING A NUMBER OF COMMON CHARACTERISTICS—UNDERDEVELOPMENT, POVERTY AND ECONOMIC DEPENDENCE OF THE FIRST TWO WORLDS.

ORIGINALLY SMALL, THE THIRD WORLD COUNTRIES HAVE NOW GROWN TO BE MORE THAN HALF OF THE WORLD'S POPULATION. BY THE BEGINNING OF THE NEXT CENTURY THEY WILL COMPOSE 80 PERCENT OF THE WORLD'S POPULATION.

I PROPOSE THAT THERE IS ALSO A THIRD WORLD IN MEDICINE, TOTALLY ANALOGOUS TO THE POLITICAL UNIVERSE. IT HAS SIMILAR CHARACTERISTICS. IT IS ESSENTIALLY "NOTHING AND WANTS TO BE SOMETHING" AND IT GENERALLY IS ASSOCIATED WITH UNDERDEVELOPMENT, POVERTY, AND

Chapter 4

The Setting

FACTORS FOR BEST POSSIBLE TALK

Although most speakers do not think much about the setting in which they will talk, experienced speakers will certainly make observations to ensure the proper conditions for their presentations.

A number of factors must be considered to ensure the best possible talk. In some instances, nothing can be done about bad situations; in others, things can be changed to increase the possibility of a good reception for the speech or the comfort of the speaker.

Lectern

A lectern must be present so that the speaker has a place to put the manuscript or notes. Trying to read a manuscript or look at notes without one will interfere with a good presentation. The lectern must also be high enough that the speaker does not have to bend over and low enough that he or she sees the audience and they can see the speaker. Speaking at an ordinary table (27 to 28 inches in height) with a manuscript lying 30 to 32 inches from your eyes will not work unless you are farsighted. It is necessary for all speakers who like or need a lectern to make sure that one is present for their talks. Be sure to ask for a lectern—a properly sized one—before starting your speech.

If you are trapped in a situation in which there is no lectern, your manuscript or notes should be held in your hand. The normal level for this would be about six inches below your line of sight while looking at the people in the first row. Look at the faces in the first row; then bring your papers up high enough to see them but not so high as to block your vision. If your notes are on cards or small papers, you may raise and lower them as needed, provided it is not such frequent movement that it distracts the audience. This enables you to drop your eyes rather than your head to see the manuscript and yet not have your face blocked out by the manuscript that is held in your hand. In any circumstance, you are much better off with a lectern.

Microphones

The proper use of the microphone is highly technical, and many books have been written about microphone technique. However, for the nonprofessional speaker who is using a microphone, there are several key suggestions. First, you must never hold the manuscript between you and your microphone. This not only hides your face from the audience, but also interferes with the voice feed into the microphone. Second, you must decide the level of voice that is satisfactory for you. Third, you must learn to keep a uniform distance from the microphone. Fourth, you must learn to evaluate your voice as it comes through the amplification system.

The level of voice you need to use will vary with the type of microphone and the size of the auditorium. You would do well to test the microphone in advance, if possible. As a general rule, you should start by using a voice level that would carry approximately twenty feet in front of you, without the microphone. Then, listening carefully to hear how effectively your voice is being carried adjust your voice volume.

While speaking, you must maintain a constant distance from the microphone. You must not rock back and forth, nor should you tilt from side to side. Some speakers have these mannerisms.

In ordinary circumstances, it may be unpleasant only to the eye, but when you use a microphone, the problems are multiplied. These habits will distort your voice going into the microphone because they cause changes in volume. You may alternately blast your audience with your voice then leave them wondering what you are saying. There is an exception to this. Again, it is primarily for experienced speakers or those who seriously practice the art. The speaker may lean into the microphone, while lowering his or her voice, to express emphasis or confidentiality. Other emotions may be expressed by pulling back from the microphone or by drawing back when the speaker wants to increase the volume of his or her voice. All of these require practice and a full realization of what you are doing. Watch a professional singer use a microphone and listen—you'll learn much.

One of the most important talents to develop for speakers who intend to do a great deal of public speaking is to be able to "hear" themselves coming back over the amplification systems so that they can learn to judge their volume and effectiveness in the use of the microphone. It is difficult to learn. However, like driving a car, once learned, it can be done automatically; while speaking, position and tone will be adjusted depending on what is heard coming back from the amplification. Because it is difficult to do and takes much practice, don't destroy your speech trying to do it while speaking for the first time. Learn to do it in your practice sessions.

When you step to the podium, look to be certain that the microphone is in a satisfactory position for your use before you start to talk. If you are inexperienced, check to see that the head of the microphone is approximately three to six inches directly in front of your mouth (or as close to that position as possible). Once you start to speak, listen to your voice coming back over the amplifying system to see if you are too close or too far from the microphone.

Lavaliere microphones (suspended from your neck) or clip-on microphones (for your tie or shirtfront or blouse front) are often available. If you are fairly rooted to the podium and do not move around much, the usual stationary microphone is probably your best bet. However, if you are a mover, if you shift positions frequently while talking or if you like to walk around during your speech, ask *in advance* for a lavaliere or a clip-on. (Don't wait until you arrive for your talk.)

A caveat: One sign of an inexperienced speaker (and you certainly do not want to appear to be one even if you are) is one who approaches the microphone and says, "Can you hear me?" A speaker should, as I indicated before, learn to hear his or her voice coming back (or know whether the microphone is on). A single tap on the microphone head prior to starting will tell you whether or not the microphone is working—and this is not always necessary.

Speakers should be warned about one more problem they may encounter with microphones. In many instances, nothing can be done about it because it is too late, but if you have the opportunity to know in advance how the room is being set up, you will be able to avoid difficulty. Unknown to most people, there are "right-handed" and "left-handed" microphones. A microphone generally extends from the lectern either on the right side or the left side as you face the audience, rarely in the middle. The difficulty occurs when the location of the projection screen forces the speaker to turn away from the microphone in order to see the screen. This occurs when the podium has a left-handed microphone and the slides are to the speaker's right (see Figure 4.1). Then the speaker either has to turn away from the slides to talk into the microphone or has to step to the left of the podium for the microphone to pick up the voice. With a right-handed microphone, this difficult maneuver is eliminated (see Figure 4.2).

So, if you have any say about setting up the room for yourself or for other speakers, be sure that the microphone is placed between the speaker and the screen, so that the speaker does not have to talk "away from" the screen, making it difficult for him

FIGURE 4.1. Incorrect Placement of Microphone and Screen

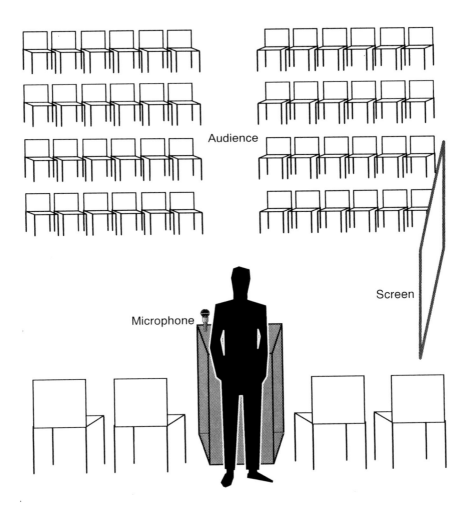

Note the left-handed microphone and right-handed screen, making it difficult to look at screen and talk into microphone.

FIGURE 4.2. Correct Placement of Microphone and Screen

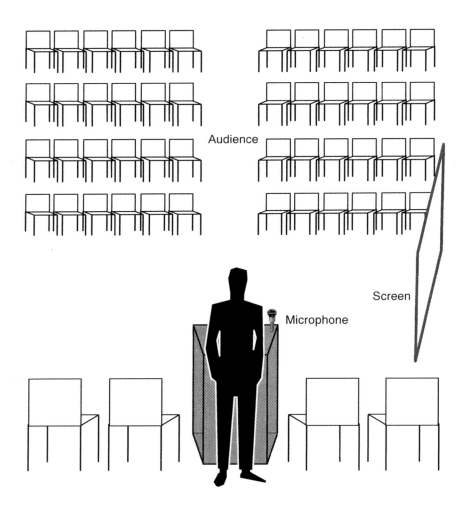

Note how a right-handed microphone and a right-handed screen eliminate the problem. This is the way a microphone should be set up in relation to a screen.

or her to see the slides. That may mean rearranging the room or changing (if possible) from a right-handed microphone to a left-handed microphone, or vice versa.

Bad amplification, a faulty microphone, or static that interferes with clear hearing will greatly annoy an audience and consequently reduce favorable reception of the speech.

Remember, if the lectern is a bad one, being too low or too high, or is in a poor location for eye contact with the audience, the speaker will be distracted and efficacy will be diminished—interfering greatly with potential success.

Environment

There are other factors in the setting that will interfere with the success of the speech. Such things as noise, smoke, a chilled room, or an overly warm room will cause problems. They interfere with an audience's concentration and attention. And if the audience isn't comfortable, your efforts—which might have been outstanding—may go down the drain. Check these physical aspects before you speak. Try to have annoying things corrected. Your audience will then be able to concentrate on what you say. Very often you may be the only one to recognize these problems or the only one with the assertiveness to do something about them.

Although it is the primary responsibility of the host organization, chairperson, or program chairperson, or all of them to prevent or correct these faults, every speaker should conduct a check before any talk. After all, if something is wrong or goes wrong, it is you the speaker who will suffer. So whenever you can do it, check in advance the physical conditions described here, as early as possible. If there is interfering noise, have it stopped. If the rostrum is too high or too low, ask for it to be corrected. But take heed; if your approach is officious or overbearing, you run the danger of being labeled obnoxious. With gentility, courtesy, and politeness, your requests will be seen as reasonable. You will be more comfortable, your audience will be more comfortable, and your talk will be much more successful.

Interruptions

What do you do if you have already started and one of these interfering factors interrupts your speech? Suppose, for example, during your talk, fire sirens sound and bells ring, but instead of passing by, they seem to stop in front of the building in which you are speaking. What do you do?

First, think about your audience. What are they imagining? Some are wondering whether there is a fire in your building. Some are wondering whether there is a fire just outside the building. Some are thinking other thoughts. However, all of them are thinking about the sirens and bells—not about your talk.

Suppose, another time, the room gets chillier and chillier. You are affected by the temperature change, and you see that members of the audience are hugging themselves, adding extra clothing if they have it, or moving about to keep warm. And no one is really listening to your talk.

In both cases, or in any similar event, stop the speech and share the problem at hand with the audience:

> Ladies and gentlemen, obviously those bells and sirens are close by. So let us stop for just a minute and check it out. Would someone please look out the window and tell us what is going on? (If it is really interesting and the group is not too large, encourage all of them to take a look.)

Once the audience has satisfied its curiosity, continue:

> You can't say that I don't bring you exciting speeches. Now, with your permission, I will continue.

Or, another possibility:

> Ladies and gentlemen, whoever is controlling the air conditioning must be working on behalf of the electric company.

Would someone (program chairperson?) please notify the engineer of our problem? In the meantime, why don't you all stand up and move about for a few minutes to get warm.

Such an approach, because it is unusual, may make some speakers (especially beginners) uncomfortable. However, let me assure you that it improves the reception of your talk every time. However, do not use it as a gimmick (which it is not) by trying to include it in every speech. That will work it to death.

Audience Fatigue

When an audience is fatigued at the beginning of your talk, or during it, you have a problem. When an audience has sat too long because of earlier parts of the program, their attention will be diminished, and their ability to concentrate on what you say will plummet. What should you do? Follow the same approach as with interruptions.

I was once an honored speaker at a national meeting. The business meeting preceding my talk dragged on twenty-five minutes past the scheduled time to start my speech. When I was finally introduced, the audience had been sitting continuously for two hours.

In this situation, my opening remark was something like this: "It's probably not a smart speaker who gives his audience a chance to get out after sitting as long as you folks have. But you deserve a break. Why not stand and stretch at your seats briefly." (Just one minute is usually sufficient to recover.)

On another occasion, I was asked to take part in a career program at a large university. There were to be three deans, each speaking about his or her own school for thirty minutes, followed by questions from the audience. The chairperson spent fifteen minutes introducing the program. The two deans who preceded me took a total of one and three-quarter hours. I was finally introduced thirty minutes after the program was to have ended.

The audience had sat continuously for the entire period of time!! My opening remark was, "I'm tired of sitting and I know you must be, too; how about standing up for a couple of minutes to get the circulation going again!" I was greeted with spontaneous applause, but more important, that audience knew I was on its side. Not one person left the room, and when they were seated again, they became interested in me. This relieved their physical fatigue that may have caused them to squirm, be uncomfortable, or possibly walk out.

These may seem like very radical things to do, and they are. I use these approaches only in extreme situations, but it is far better to use them than to try to compete with something which has completely drawn your audience's attention away from you or which interferes so much that your audience will not hear you or listen to you. Don't compete, cooperate. If your audience isn't comfortable, they won't hear a word you say.

Chapter 5

The Speaker

The key to any successful talk is the speaker. To be successful, the speaker must first have specific reasons for giving the talk—objectives for the speech.

SPEECH OBJECTIVES

You as a speaker should approach your audience with four major objectives in mind:

- To be heard
- To be understood
- To be believed
- To move the audience to action

The first three are clear, but in professional talks, "to move the audience to action" may more properly be to move them to accept and believe in your ideas, theories, or proposals—whether it's your particular approach to a problem or a new diagnosis or therapy.

Achieving these objectives will depend on how you approach your audience and how you convince them. A number of factors will play a role: speaking with authority, developing the ability to communicate, and using all modes of expressiveness.

The first, authority of the speaker, provides recognition that gives him or her the force to be convincing. Such authority may precede the speaker by virtue of status, title, or reputation.

However, in most instances, a speaker is not nationally known and must earn authority by exhibiting command of the subject or by poise on the platform that gives him or her an aura of authority. (Warning: always be careful that you do not confuse authority with pomposity; this will turn your audience off.)

The speaker who appears to be immersed in the subject will be more likely to achieve the speech objectives. The speaker must convince the audience that he or she believes in the material being presented. If a speaker comes across to the audience as an authority, he or she will have an easier time "selling" them. However, more than one speaker has taken the platform with indisputable credentials, only to destroy credibility with a miserable speech.

The ability of the speaker to communicate will also help determine effect on the audience. Does the speaker talk down or communicate? Does the speaker drive relentlessly for audience response? Is the speaker interested in the audience and what the audience gets from the presentation or is he or she only interested in finishing the presentation and getting off the platform?

Vocal expressiveness is another important factor—timing, range, pauses, phrasing. These will be discussed in a later chapter.

GESTURES AND ANIMATION

Perhaps one of the most controversial areas in all of public speaking, and particularly in professional speaking, is that of physical expressiveness, the use of movement and gestures. For some unexplainable reason, people, particularly in science, have developed the attitude that the more formal, stiff, unrelaxed, and rigid they are on the platform, the more scientific their presentation is, believing that animation reduces the audience's acceptance of their accuracy. In fact, scientific and professional people often carry this philosophy into their writing. In neither instance does stiffness make the presentation more scientific.

Animation contributes a great deal to the success of any speech, technical or otherwise. As a speaker, you should feel free to move about the platform, depending on your own needs, preferences, and the physical circumstances. You must be comfortable with what you do. Your movements should not be so dramatic as to distract attention from what you are saying, but on the other hand, you need not remain rooted to one spot, motionless throughout your talk, as has been taught in so many public speaking courses.

Movement should be spontaneous and natural. You do not have to be rigid or move with the stiffness of a robot; your posture should be relaxed but not slouched or informal.

Gestures do add a measure of animation, but if the use of gestures does not come to you naturally, you must spend considerable time polishing this aspect of your speaking by practicing the development of natural gestures. Gestures for the beginner should be well thought out but should appear very natural and be used as seasoning—enough to give flavor to the meat (of the talk) but not so much that it overpowers the taste.

Your facial expressions should reflect what you are saying, and they will, if you believe in what you are saying. If you are delivering a happy, funny, or interesting thought, your appearance should project that. If your commentary is sad or serious, you expression should match. Your interest in the subject and your excitement about it (which you should have) should show in your facial expressions and your gestures.

Gestures are a "must" for any speaker who wants to be interesting. I have described the extreme of standing rigid without gestures, but the other extreme should also be avoided—being unaware that you are overusing gestures and body movements. One of the most enlightening methods of studying body movements and gestures is to watch television with the sound turned down to observe closely the gestures and body movements of the people who are speaking, without the distraction of the spoken voice. It is especially instructive to do this with news broadcasts, in which the anchorperson is limited in movement but still generally manages to use expressive appearance, animation, and gestures to spice the presentation without detracting from it.

INTERFERING FACTORS

There are numerous factors that may interfere and possibly spoil your speech. You owe it to yourself and your audience to be in the best possible condition and the most comfortable state for your talk. As a speaker (or potential speaker), you must take these factors into consideration to succeed in presenting a medical talk.

Overindulgence and fatigue are among the internal factors that may interfere with a speaker's performance. Overeating prior to the meeting may cause enough discomfort for the speaker to affect a presentation—and it is most apt to occur to an after-dinner (or luncheon) speaker. Many professionals prefer to have a very light snack an hour or two before the meeting (or dinner) to avoid being hungry and overeating. At the banquet, they "play" with the food to appear to be eating. They arrange to have dinner after the banquet, if they are hungry, enabling them to speak without being uncomfortable. Others prefer to eat lightly from the food served. The same generalizations apply to midafternoon or early evening speeches at which food is served. Take it easy. Don't overeat. Stay comfortable.

The same advice is obviously applicable to overindulgence, or indulgence at all, in alcohol. This commentary will not be an antialcohol campaign. However, there are two precautions. First, the effects of alcohol are well known. Even small amounts can decrease the user's sharpness and should never be allowed to interfere with the effectiveness of a talk. Second, any speaking faults you show or errors you make in your presentation, however small, may be blamed on the alcohol. If you as a speaker are seen with a drink in your hand prior to your address, people will be apt to blame the alcohol for any mistakes or hesitations or anything they do not like about your talk. My strong recommendation: Do not drink alcohol prior to delivering a speech.

Fatigue, another internal factor, will greatly decrease the speaker's efficiency and effectiveness. It is necessary to be as well rested as the circumstances will permit. Some noted speakers have been criticized as aloof because they do not make themselves available for conferences or socialization prior to a talk. But if this kind of activity is tiring to the speaker, it should be avoided, even at the expense of being thought of as slightly stuffy; after all, the speech is the reason the speaker is there—and that must be successful. Socialization can take place after the talk.

EYE CONTACT

The speaker must alway maintain as much eye contact with the audience as possible. After all, in one-on-one conversations, the most effective communicators are the ones with sincere and prolonged eye contact. Various suggestions have been made for beginners who are uncomfortable looking at audience members and talking to them. It has been recommended by some "teachers" of public speaking that the speaker should find one person's eyes in the audience and speak directly to him or her throughout the talk. Others have recommended picking a spot on the wall behind or about the level of the listeners' heads and speak to that spot.

Neither of these suggestions are great advice, even though starting with them may relieve some of the speaker's anxiety. Although it is true that as a speaker you should speak directly to individuals in your audience, it is best done by shifting your eyes from one audience member to another audience member, speaking phrases or sentences to each one in turn. You do not have to look at everyone in the audience, but in time, you will gradually learn to recognize receptive and friendly faces in the audience. When you are able to do this, it is wise for you to look around the room, pick out these faces, and look at them. Then speak to them as you would speak to any friend, eye to eye, while communicating your message directly to them (and the rest of your audience).

Remember, it is a two-way street: you expect the audience to look at you, and therefore, you should look at the audience. Moreover, if your speech is to be successful, you must survey your audience, judge their reactions to your talk by observing their faces and their body language, and make any adjustments that are necessary to preserve the integrity of your speech.

NERVOUSNESS

A word should be said about nervousness. Almost no speaker is completely free of nervousness. Almost everyone, no matter how experienced, has some degree of butterflies before beginning a performance. The great actress Helen Hayes, a veteran of thousands of stage appearances, once said that a performer who doesn't get a little apprehensive before going on does not really care about the audience.

If you have the opportunity sometime, watch a professional before he or she approaches the microphone or goes on the stage. Practically all of them have little nervous mannerisms—adjusting a tie, clearing the throat, or a number of other things. So if the best speakers do it, don't feel bad because you do.

One of the ways for the beginner to reduce nervousness is to practice relaxation while being introduced. This means relaxing your head and neck muscles by thinking consciously about doing so. Deep breathing will also help, but beware of hyperventilation. One of the best techniques for the speaker upon reaching the podium is to take a couple of deep breaths before starting the talk to become well-oxygenated, and at the same time, relieve some anxiety. This pause is part of the "focal pause" discussed in the next chapter. However, take care not to become "breathless" and sound as though you have just run up a flight of steps.

Chapter 6

The Talk

Every talk must have three parts: the *introduction* or *opening*, the *central theme* or *body*, and the *conclusion* or *summary*. As I was taught in my early days in debating in college, first tell them what you are going to say, say it, then tell them what you've said.

THE OPENING

When introduced, the speaker must not rush to the podium, but must not dawdle, either. The speaker should approach the podium deliberately, pause, look at the audience, and perhaps smile. This is called the focal pause because it gives the audience a chance to look at the speaker—focus on him or her—and gives the speaker a chance to adjust before beginning the talk. It also gives more impact to the first words of the presentation.

Many speakers experience great anxiety about their talks, and I often feel that the anxiety peaks during the introduction and for a few moments afterward. In some cases, speakers may actually begin to talk (or "chat") on the way to the podium; they do this out of nervousness and inability to endure silence. But this is wrong. Speakers must follow the *focal pause* procedure.

The opening of any talk should be an icebreaker, something to gain the audience's attention. It should be interesting or startling or humorous so that it will "grab" the listener immediately. This is important because it may set the tone for maintaining the listeners' attention and interest and may determine whether the audience will really listen to the remainder of your speech. An icebreaker should be short and never left to chance. It is far too important. Inexperienced speakers would be well advised to prepare each opening carefully and rehearse it assiduously, almost to the point of memory.

Inexperienced speakers should also be warned: never begin with an apology. There is no place for "I really didn't want to give this talk, but there was no one else available," or "I hope you'll bear with me, I don't particularly like this subject," or any of the other hackneyed apologies that are so frequently used by the unsophisticated or the insecure.

To begin, the speaker gives a salutation, depending on the group being addressed. In the past few years, long and formal salutations have become less popular. Once, all speeches had to start with acknowledgement of every distinguished presence in the audience or on the platform and all the officers of the group. Speakers would say, "Mr. Chairman, Reverend Clergy, Madame Secretary, Distinguished Platform Guests, and Ladies and Gentlemen." Today, much less of this is being done. I personally prefer to limit salutations to the bare minimum or use none at all.

At this point, it would be proper, if the speaker can do it, to ad lib an appropriate remark (which might be either funny or serious and would refer to the particular occasion) to some previous comments that were made or to some occurrence or experience that the speaker and the audience share. It might be a comment on your introduction, the chairperson's remarks, or something that happened just before your talk.

It is important that the remark tie in with something that the audience can recognize. A beautiful example occurred on a Jerry Lewis Muscular Dystrophy Telethon, broadcast from Caesar's Palace in Las Vegas. Viewers of these programs will recall the pattern—entertainment by superstars interspersed with serious messages about muscular dystrophy. Following a well-received song by Frank Sinatra, Jerry Lewis introduced a young minister recently stricken with the disease. Jerry welcomed him, and in response, the minister said, "Jerry, this is quite an honor. I am probably the only clergyman to appear on stage at Caesar's Palace and have Frank Sinatra as his opening act." His spontaneous wit earned him one of the best laughs of the day—and the immediate interest and respect of the audience.

If you have the talent to create interesting ad libs, you are already ahead. If not, prepare them. Often ad libs given by experienced speakers are really well rehearsed and have been used many times before. However, they are made to sound spontaneous.

Following this, the speaker may proceed in one of several ways: using humor very carefully, telling an illustrative story or anecdote, making a startling statement, asking arresting questions, or explaining why this topic is important to the audience. The speaker then should give a brief preview of what will be discussed in the talk.

The icebreaker may fit into any one of the categories previously described. On the other hand, it may take an entirely different form. I personally have copied methods used by a number of noted speakers in the past. I very frequently tell a prepared joke that relates to my topic or the occasion. When I am able to come up with a suitable ad lib (either funny or merely appropriate), I will usually use that just before or just after the joke.

Appropriateness is the key word in choosing any of this material. One of my favorite openings is the following (using these words immediately upon reaching the podium):

Driving here this evening, I could not help but think about the world-famous neurosurgeon in Philadelphia. In his older years, he spent a great deal of time traveling about the country, to talk about his field of specialty. He always went to the local meetings in his own car, driven by a chauffeur. One evening, he was driving from Philadelphia to Lancaster on the Pennsylvania Turnpike and said to his chauffeur, "Charles, are you coming in to hear my talk tonight?" The chauffeur thought for a moment and then said, "No, sir, I'm not." And after a brief pause he added, "In fact, I've heard your talk so much I think I can give it myself. In fact, I think I can give it as well as you do." The doctor perked up and said, "Oh, you do, do you? Well let's see about that." So they stopped at the next turnpike restaurant; the doctor put on the chauffeur's uniform, and the chauffeur put on the doctor's pin-striped suit. From there they proceeded to the hospital where the doctor was scheduled to speak. Sure enough, the chauffeur in the doctor's suit gave the doctor's speech, and he gave it well. At the end he was greeted with tumultuous applause, and as it died down, a physician in the front row raised his hand and asked a technical question. Not to be stumped, the chauffeur in the doctor's suit looked at the questioner and said, "Sir that's a dumb question. That's the dumbest question I have ever heard. In fact, it is so dumb, I'm going to let my chauffeur answer it." I want you to know that's why I brought Charlie Brown (someone who has accompanied me, another speaker on the program, the chairperson, or someone known to the audience) with me. If you have any questions at the end of my talk, he'll be happy to answer them.

In my medical speaking classes, I conduct a class exercise in which the students are required to prepare in writing a satisfactory opening (and closing) for a medical talk. One student came up with an excellent icebreaker by using a startling statement (again, these are the speaker's first words):

Look around. One out of every seven of you is or will become an alcoholic.

Don't you think that line stopped the audience in its tracks? Don't you think every member of that audience wanted to hear what he had to say? Don't you think the speaker had them in the palm of his hand? You bet he did, and he could go on to develop his talk about alcoholism and its ramifications.

THE BODY

The body of the talk must be well organized. It must be logical, understandable, and never, at any time, convoluted. The body of an average talk should contain anywhere from two to five major headings. More than this is too much for an audience to retain and appreciate during the normal length talk. If more than this is needed, perhaps it is best to use a handout for the audience. Actually, a speaker probably is better off with only two or three major headings.

In introducing each new heading, it is wise for the speaker to review the headings already covered. A simple review is sufficient: "Now that you have some insight into the pathogenesis and symptoms of rheumatic fever, let me discuss some of the dilemmas of diagnosis." It does not have to be a mechanical, "I have presented pathogenesis and symptoms; now I will discuss diagnosis." Note the smoother flow of the first example.

Very little space will be devoted to a discussion of the body of the talk. From my observations, this is the area that needs the least amount of instruction; almost all professionals can manage to outline this part of a talk and do it satisfactorily. It is the "trimmings" to which our discussions are really dedicated.

The varieties of outlining the body are endless and often depend on the subject matter. For example, in medical topics, the simplest and the most trite is to use the following:

1. Etiology (with three or four causes)
2. Diagnosis (five or six high points of diagnosis)
3. Treatment (listing the treatments available)

Some talks must, by their nature, follow this kind of pattern, but a talk can be made much more interesting if the speaker can find a better way to approach the same material. One of my colleagues was charged with putting together a course in medical history. As everyone knows, there appears to be only one way to teach this: You start with ancient Greece, trace medicine through the Roman Empire, and continue on up until modern day. You divide the time periods into convenient sections, according to how many hours of teaching you have to do. Not this professor. He decided that history was really alive and could be made interesting to students. He therefore took nine topics (for a nine-hour course) and traced the development of each one through eons of history. What made this approach effective was that he chose such subjects as wound healing, pregnancy and abortion, and other similar interesting topics. Through them, he was teaching history.

The speaker knows best what message he or she wants to develop and will make the outline accordingly—again with the warning that no more than five major points should be made in any one speech, although subtopics may be discussed.

THE CONCLUSION

The conclusion, like the opening, is far too important to be left to chance and must be very carefully prepared. First, a brief summary should be given of what has been said in the body of the talk, and should be more expository than merely mechanical repetition. Then, there should be some sort of powerful statement, a finale—preferably something that will tie in with the introduction, the body of the talk, or the day's theme—something appropriate that your audience can relate to. It might be humor, a poem, or a quotation. It might be a strong statement, an illustration, a story, or a call to action or an outlook for the future.

Inexperienced speakers often ask whether this kind of conclusion is not too contrived and whether it is possible to give a good scientific speech and at the same time provide a powerful ending. A perfect example is a splendid article on smoking, which appeared in the *American Journal of Public Health,* titled "Pro Bono Publico" (for the good of the public). This article surveyed the smoking habits of people in Durham, North Carolina, and viewed those habits in light of the city's being a tobacco center. The article received its title because, as indicated in its opening paragraph, the first smoking tobacco manufactured in America was called "Pro Bono Publico." The final paragraph is a natural—a twist of language that is its own haymaker:

> In a recent visit by one of us . . . to a Durham tobacco factory where regular guided tours are a popular tourist and local attraction, three cigarettes were handed out to all comers. Visitors were told that each employee received a free pack of cigarettes daily, a whole carton on special holidays and free access to rejected cigarettes. How much such practices contribute to the smoking patterns and mortality rates described in this article it is not possible to say, but perhaps Pro Bono Publico has now become at least from the standpoint of health, Pro Malo Publico. (Green and Sabler, 1977, p. 738)

What a powerful ending for as scholarly an article as you can get! And, this is in a scientific publication, more formal and circumspect than almost all oral presentations. What a great example of good medical writing.

Of course you can use a powerful haymaker to end your talk and not lose one iota of scientific respectability. The real problem is that most of us do not say it this well and most cannot express it so powerfully.

THANKS

Although it may seem polite for a speaker, at the end of the talk, to say "Thank you" to the audience or to say "Thank you for your kind attention," these have become so hackneyed and meaningless that they should be eliminated. Not only is it poor style because it is trite, but even more, it is usually a trail-off—the dropping of the speaker's voice as the talk is ended. It greatly diminishes the impact of the speaker's carefully crafted (hopefully) finale. The trail-off "Thank you" is generally a crutch used by speakers who are not quite sure how to end the speech or leave the platform. It equates with saying, "I'm finished." I would recommend that a speaker never use these expressions.

Not for every routine speech and not for every presentation, but there are times when a speaker wants to, and should, express appreciation to the audience or to the organization that invited him or her. When? This is completely up to the speaker to decide. It may be an honor lecture or a talk following an award. It may be that the speaker has been singled out for this talk. Whatever the reason, it is solely in the judgment of the speaker to make this decision. Once the speaker has decided, however, then the expression of thanks takes on importance and significance and should never be limited to the usual dull, emotionless, half-mumbled "Thank you" described before. The expression of appreciation, when deemed necessary, should be a full one, given either at the beginning of the talk or at the end. It should name the organization and be a sincere expression of gratitude. For example:

> Before I present to you some of my experiences in my research on hypertension, I must pause to express my deepest appreciation to the Pennsylvania Society of Hypertension Research for inviting me to be the featured speaker at this special program. I am grateful to you, and I thank you for the opportunity.

Please note, however, that I would use something such as this after giving my icebreaker introduction. First, get their attention. Then, say what you want to—in this case, your thanks.

Or, express your thanks in your closing:

> I cannot conclude my remarks without offering a note of gratitude. I want to thank Dr. Carl Benjamin, your program chairman, and the entire College of Music Therapy, for inviting me to be your banquet speaker. The honor is mine, and I want you to know I appreciate it.

Again, I would use this just before the finale, the haymaker, the vigorous closing. However, even though it might be improved with a stronger closing added, it could stand by itself as an adequate ending, if delivered with a strong voice and conviction.

Note how much stronger these expressions of thanks are and how they have become personalized. Also, in this form it cannot be mumbled under your breath and sound like an afterthought. It is specific. It is a strong ending. If you want to express your thanks, be strong and say it right.

A trail-off, as I have indicated, can ruin a perfectly good presentation. Instead of creating a strong ending, the trail-off fades down into nothingness. There are trail-offs other than the weak "Thank you": a speaker who rifles through his pages or searches his notes and says "I think I finished what I have to say," "That's probably the end of my talk," or "I think I'd better stop here." The audience is entitled to a speaker who knows when the talk is finished, has completed what needed to be said, and is sufficiently prepared that he or she recognizes reaching the end of the talk without having to fumble through these weaselley words (or papers). As with introductions, there almost never should be an apology, except in the rare instance of a gross malfeasance, such as arriving seriously late or speaking for over the time limit. Trail-offs are often bumbling apologies for miniscule occurrences because the speaker does not know how else to conclude his or her talk.

The posture of authority—which you want to maintain for strength in your presentation—demands that you end your talk firmly and with conviction. You should leave the platform with the same air of authority with which you started your speech. That means saying the final words of your speech (as prepared in advance), with conviction, saying them so that they are fully heard, picking up your notes or papers if you have any (without fumbling around), and leaving the podium with dignity and returning to your seat. Reminder: authority is not pomposity.

TIME LIMITS

The bending of time limits by the speaker is, in general, to be condemned. Every talk has a time limit. Sometimes that limit is published, as with a printed program (which indicates the time of starting and the time of ending), or by instruction from the organization or program chairperson. Going over that time limit is an insult to those who invited you as well as to the audience. It may also be an indication that you do not know how to prepare a talk properly. Almost no one has a message so important that he or she has the right to talk thirty minutes when invited to speak for fifteen. Every speech should fit the time slot assigned, or the speaker should not accept the assignment.

If you are honored by an invitation to give a talk, you have the obligation of preparing carefully, choosing the most important things to say, and keeping within the time frame assigned. This requires careful preparation of the material as well as timing of the talk. A speaker should also be able to control digressions from the prepared talk so that it does not go overtime and to be able to end the talk at the appropriate time, even though all the prepared material may not have been covered. The more experience you get as a speaker, the more capable you should become at doing this.

What do you do if someone has encroached on your starting time and you are beginning your talk late? This is a difficult question to answer and one that depends on where you are, who you are, and what you are talking about. I personally believe—and there are those who disagree—that the speaker should attempt to finish at the scheduled time, even if it means cutting his own material short. Let's look at some examples:

- You are scheduled for your presentation from 10:00 to 10:30. Because of circumstances, you are not introduced until 10:05. Under these conditions, I would shorten my speech by five minutes, leaving out some of the less important details, and I would attempt to wind down as close to 10:30 as possible. This will be noted by the program chairperson and the audience. Both will be appreciative.
- You are scheduled to speak from 11:15 to 12:00. Because of others' mistakes, you do not reach the podium until 11:35. Sure, your talk is important and deserving of forty-five minutes. Sure, the audience is entitled to hear your entire speech. However, you are approaching lunch hour. According to the printed program (which you presume the entire audience has read), you will finish at noon. At noon, or just a few minutes after, your audience will begin to look at their watches. They are starting to get hungry. They will become restless, and the longer you go on, the more restless they will become. The effectiveness of your talk diminishes through this period of restlessness, and you lose your audience's attention. In this situation, attempt to shorten your speech so that you finish exactly at noon, or if beyond that, only a few minutes.

What if the program is so late that there is no reasonable expectation of your presenting your speech condensed to simply a few minutes? You simply have to wing it. You might ask the program chairperson what he or she would like to do. You might ask whether there is more time available a little later. You might ask the audience whether they want you to continue and offer to understand if anyone wishes to leave early. This allows for a more comfortable audience, one which knows you are concerned about them and their sitting power.

Perhaps it is wiser for the speaker to prepare the material so that the talk will fall just short of the allotted time, rather than preparing to fill every second of the scheduled time, unless he or she is an experienced speaker who can time the talk as it moves along. The speaker might even prepare some "swing" material that can be used if more time needs to be filled or can be easily eliminated if unneeded. This helps a beginning speaker to adjust to fluctuations of time.

Concern for the audience is a major consideration. I am not merely suggesting some act of altruism: it is also very selfish to be concerned because an uncomfortable audience will lose most of the points you have to make. Showing that you care about your audience and realizing that they must be comfortable if they are going to absorb anything, will win audiences for you.

Chapter 7

Voice and Delivery

DELIVERING THE TALK

Delivery of a talk is the translating of symbols into meaningful thoughts; it is not translating them into words. The error made by most beginning speakers is to read words rather than thoughts. Reading words results in choppy and unintelligible delivery. With proper delivery techniques, you tell the audience how to understand the words you are saying. In discussing each of these attributes of voice and making suggestions for delivering the talk, I will attempt to include recommendations for marking your manuscript, in case you are going to read, to give valuable instructions to yourself in delivering the talk. This is in line with what was suggested in the chapter on "Preparing the Manuscript."

To understand the difference between delivering words and delivering thoughts, read each word below with exactly the same monotonous emphasis:

Jack-and-Jill-went-up-the-hill-to-fetch-a-pail-of-water-Jack-fell-down-and-broke-his-crown-and-Jill-came-tumbling-after.

Or (reading line by line):

Jack and Jill went up the hill
to fetch a pail of water.

    Jack fell down and broke his crown,
    and Jill came tumbling after.

Here we have grouped words into thoughts, added punctuation (even verbally), and made it much more listenable.

    There are a number of attributes of the voice that you can use, with some practice and training, to improve your delivery. These matters usually concern singers more than speakers, although they were emphasized years ago in speaking, when students were taught elocution. Study of these attributes is generally not for beginners in speech or for occasional speakers, but serious students of public speaking might profit from studying them. They are presented here for completeness of our discussion, not to confuse the beginners. Novices can wait until they have more experience, but they certainly can profit from thinking about them.

Emphasis

    This helps to communicate ideas. For example, the sentence, "I think he is the guilty man," can vary with the reading. Try reading it aloud seven times, each time putting emphasis on a different word. First "I," then "think" and so on. Note that each emphasis changes the meaning of the sentence. In preparing the manuscript, one way to attract your attention to the emphasis you want to make is to underline in advance what words you need to stress. You may even choose to use one, two, or three underlines, depending on what prominence you intend to give to any particular thought or word. Using our previous example, the manuscript might read:

    I think he is the guilty man.

or

    I *think* he is the guilty man.

or

I think *he* is the guilty man.

All of these statements have different meanings. Underlining saves you the agony of making a decision while in the middle of your talk or trying to remember which meaning you intended.

Phrasing

Phrasing is a very complex use of words, achieved by regrouping them into subtle changes of meaning, and there are many nuances to achieving proper phrasing. Many people have natural phrasing ability—an example is the outstanding phrasing of Frank Sinatra, which many think is the quality responsible for much of his success as a singer. In phrasing, some help may be given by the use of commas, periods, and paragraphs. These are natural stops for people, but they do not necessarily reflect the best possible phrasing for oral delivery.

In preparing your talk, decide in advance how you want to phrase your important sentences or thoughts. Then mark your manuscript: indicate a brief stop as a single slash between words, a longer stop with a double slash, and a prolonged stop with a triple slash. For a good example of phrasing, read the lines from *The Tempest* below, first reading it line by line as a grade school child might read a poem. You will find that the words have very little meaning read that way. Then read it with proper phrasing, using the punctuation that Shakespeare used and notice the difference in meaning.

> Full fathom five thy father lies;
> of his bones are coral made;
> Those are pearls that were his eyes:
> Nothing of him doth fade
> But doth suffer a sea-change

Into something rich and strange.
Sea-nymphs hourly ring his knell:
Ding-Dong!
Hark! Now I hear them—ding, dong, bell!

Now look at the same lines marked up for personal phrasing by using slashes as described previously:

Full fathom five / thy father lies; //
   of his bones are coral made; //
Those are pearls / that were his eyes: //
   Nothing of him / doth fade
But doth suffer a sea-change /
Into something rich and strange.///
Sea-nymphs hourly / ring his knell:
Ding-Dong!
Hark! / Now I hear them / —ding, / dong, / bell!

With the manuscript marks, you do not have to remember how you wanted to say it.

Pitch

The pitch of the voice gives widely varied meanings to the words that are spoken. First, every speaker should be aware of the pitch of his or her own voice. Some speakers have high-pitched voices that may come across as whiny. Others have deep basso profundo voices. All speakers should listen to themselves on tape a number of times and then attempt to change the pitch of their usual speaking voice to a well-modulated middle-of-the-road pitch, appropriate for most speaking. From the normal tone, speakers should learn to modulate their voice to the thoughts being expressed. The pitch should depend on what they are trying to convey. High-pitched voices, in general, convey excitement, fear, anger, intensity of conviction, gaiety, and alarm.

Low-pitched voices reflect reverence, awe, respect, and disdain. Try using your voice to express these emotions and see how they correlate. Neophyte speakers would be wise to mark on their manuscripts where they intend to raise or lower the pitch of their voice by using a curved arrow pointing upward or downward— or some similar sign of their own choosing so that it will alert them to the pitch change.

> I am glad John came along.
> He is the most determined man I know.

Lower the pitch of the voice (as the arrow indicates just before "He"), conveying a feeling of awe in the second sentence.

Pace

The usual pace of most speakers may have to be adjusted for oral reading. In general, unsophisticated speakers, out of nervousness, talk too quickly and may have to slow down. On the other hand, when it involves reading a manuscript, the speaker may read too slowly and have to speed up the pace. The normal pace should be somewhere between 150 to 180 words per minute or about two and a half minutes to read a double-spaced page of type. Try practicing reading at this pace, using a watch to time yourself. A rapid pace suggests to the listener fear, indignation, joy, and animation, whereas a slow pace indicates assurance, calm, dignity, reverence, or despair. Try the different paces and note your associated feelings. For marking up the manuscript as a reminder, the beginning writer may want to put a capital F, S, or M—representing, fast, slow, or medium—in the left-hand margin. Others prefer to put such signals directly into the script over the lines to which they apply. If the passage requiring special pacing is longer than a few words, it might be wise to set it off in the manuscript as a separate line or lines, for example:

When examining a child's belly, the physician should take care to <u>move slowly and easily and gently</u> if he is to be able to make a good diagnosis.

or

When examining a child's belly, the physician should take care to move

slowly and easily and gently if he is to be able to make a good diagnosis.

Voice Volume (Loudness)

Volume changes send different meanings to the listener and should be used with great care. Increases in volume give special emphasis to the words being said; sometimes they convey anger, argumentativeness, conviction, or enthusiasm. On the other hand, decreasing the volume also creates emphasis and tells the listener of sincerity, self-confidence, and confidentiality.

It is interesting that a dramatic drop in the volume of your voice will often get more attention and make for greater emphasis than shouting. Often, angry or upset teachers will get a faster response from their classes by lowering their voices almost to a whisper.

The manuscript should be marked "louder" or "softer"; some speakers prefer to use a color index for volume, perhaps red or green. However, it is important to decide how *you* want to indicate volume to emphasize your thoughts and to mark your script accordingly.

There are other ways of controlling what the voice implies, but most of these belong in voice-training manuals rather than in public speaking for professionals. *Punch* is a staccato way of delivering words rapid-fire for special emphasis. The best example of punch is the hard sell of certain disc jockeys and television salesmen, in which every word is emphasized and delivered in a loud and very rapid form. A *drawl,* or slowing of the speech, very often creates the impression of indecision or indifference. A *harsh* voice may be used to indicate displeasure or resentment, and *whispers* may be used as special emphasis or to indicate weakness, illness, tenderness, or caution. When used to give emphasis, as I have said, it is amazing that the softer the words are spoken, the more emphatic they become to the listener.

Voice control and manipulation by these or other methods may seem a complicated subject to those not directly interested in voice, but its effectiveness in speaking from the platform cannot be overemphasized.

A good example of the difference voice control makes can be found in the use of the word "Oh." Try this exercise: say this one word to express, in order:

- Anger
- Curiosity
- Surprise
- Ambivalence
- Pleasure
- Enthusiasm

See if you can say the same word to convey these different meanings to an audience.

The speaker must be aware that many of the things he or she says can change meaning to the listener, depending on the emphasis and the use of the speaker's voice. If you want to get the proper meaning across to the audience, you must plan the use of your voice.

The Pause

The advertising profession has always had a profound respect for the use of white space in an advertisement. Rarely is high quality attributed to advertisements that pack every single piece of space with copy and pictures, a jumble of type, and illustration known as "borax." Borax does sell for certain kinds of businesses, but award-winning advertising shows a great deal of white space, particularly the intelligent use of such space.

The pause in a talk is the white space of an advertisement. Used properly it provides strong emphasis and proper pacing for the talk.

Pauses, even beyond the ones usually indicated in the manuscript by punctuation, should be used intelligently throughout a talk. However, unsophisticated speakers have a nervous fear of silence. You may be fearful that the audience will interpret your pause as your inability to continue. You may think that they will be uncomfortable because of the quiet. You may be personally uncomfortable or upset by the silence. This is what causes some people to say, "Uhh" every time they pause to convert to a new thought. It also accounts, in part, for the repetitive "Ya know," used so frequently by today's youth.

Think about yourself in a one-on-one situation with a person you have met just recently. Think about the difficulty in producing "small talk" and think about what "small talk" is. It is a method of filling up quiet time—or pauses—so that neither of the parties feels uncomfortable, stupid, or unsocial. Now visualize yourself with your mate, an old friend, or someone very close. You are comfortable with pauses; you are comfortable with breaks in conversation. Neither party panics because there is a "lull" in the conversation.

Although a pause in a talk may seem an eternity to an inexperienced speaker, it rarely lasts more than two or three seconds. A deliberate pause may be used for emphasis, to allow time for a message or thought to sink into the minds of the audience, to allow the speaker to breathe, or for any other purpose the speaker desires.

In the manuscript, suspension points (. . .) or the use of a special color slash might remind the speaker where he or she wants the special pause or pauses to take place.

IS IT ACTING?

Experienced speakers are often asked whether public speaking is merely acting. The reader, looking closely at some of the suggestions in this book, and especially at this section on voice, might well ask the same question. One wise professor of public speaking said, in answer to this question, "Act human or don't act at all." This is as good advice as anyone can give to the beginning speaker. It is true that some professional speakers may go to an extreme and develop acting styles, enhancing their presentation or turning off audiences if they overdo it. But what you call it is not important; if attention to some additional details improves your presentation and increases receptivity of the audience, do it.

Sincerity and Enthusiasm

These two qualities are the most important for guaranteeing the success of the speaker. Without these—even using all the other suggestions—your speech is only mediocre and generally unconvincing.

Improper grammar, unmarked manuscripts, untrained voice, and all the other faults speakers may have are surely to be avoided, but these will take on decreased importance if the speaker conveys to the audience sincerity and enthusiasm about the subject. And the feelings must be real. This does more to convince an audience and to have them remember what you say than any other single thing that you can do. Sincerity and enthusiasm are conveyed to the audience in several ways, including body movements and use of the voice, face, and gestures. All of these must be well controlled and well coordinated to convey these emotions.

IMPROVING YOUR TALK

Nothing is more valuable to a beginning speaker than to get feedback from a good critic. "Good" in this sense primarily means honest, one who will truthfully report likes and dislikes about your speech. Of course, it is best to get your critique from someone who is experienced and knowledgeable about professional speaking or public speaking. However, in the absence of an expert, a good honest spouse or close friend will be very helpful.

Whenever possible a speaker should record the talk on tape and listen to it several times, whether reading a script or talking extemporaneously. After listening carefully and observing errors, he or she should then re-record the speech. This is analagous to what you do when you edit a paper for publication.

Chapter 8

Reading a Speech

In reading a speech, eye contact with the audience should be maintained at least 60 percent of the time. With less contact than this, the effectiveness of your communication is lost.

Reading should be done by maintaining your head in a relatively normal position (facing your audience) and lowering and raising your eyes—lowering them to grasp a phrase or two and raising them to deliver those ideas. Your head should not go up and down; it should move very little. This process can be impeded if the physical conditions at the podium are less than perfect, as described in Chapter 4. There is a tendency among beginning speakers to "put their noses in the manuscript" and read.

The speaker should look at the manuscript, take in a thought or phrase, look up at the audience, and repeat that same thought or phrase—even if he or she makes a mistake in one or two of the words. Whenever it is possible in the manuscript, the thought or phrase should be written on a single line, and the manuscript should be written so that each line is a single thought or phrase unto itself. The manuscript in its first copy should be marked for this arrangement then retyped so that the speaker can recognize this readily. Every manuscript to be read must be edited for speaking.

Do not read words, only ideas. Reading words becomes singsong and boring, and you will lose listeners in very short order. Go back and reread Jack and Jill. In order to perfect this technique, you must read the manuscript several times; your ability to transmit broad ideas will in part depend on your reading skills.

IMPROVING YOUR READING

The aim of any program for improving the speaker's ability to read a manuscript is to give him or her the appearance and sound of being extemporaneous. Our best examples are TV and radio performers who read from manuscripts or sometimes from tele-prompters, yet appear to be spontaneous. A number of techniques will offer the inexperienced speaker some help.

Beginners should read aloud anything they can get their hands on. Particularly helpful will be texts that are not written for oral presentation because these are so much more difficult. If you can master them, you will be better able to master a talk written for oral presentation. Newspapers have been recommended by some authorities as excellent sources for practice readings because if you can read the closely printed columns of the newspaper and give them the proper emphasis you will have mastered the art. It has been said occasionally in praise of an actor that he could read a menu or the telephone book and make it sound interesting. That's an unreachable goal, but an inspirational one.

Practicing your particular talk will also be helpful. Every speech should be rehearsed several times so that you are well acquainted with it, especially with the sound of it when spoken aloud.

A good way to start is to divide your paper into sections. Ask a friend or relative to help you. Tell him or her what you are specifically going to say in each section, then read it aloud until your listener clearly gets the message you have described. No one is too talented or too brilliant to neglect practicing the reading of a new script in advance. Or, you could practice reading your manuscript aloud until your friend is able to give a clear summary of what you are saying.

One of the difficulties in reading a long manuscript is that the speaker very often has a tendency to fall asleep mentally while doing it. That means the speaker is "mouthing" words—they hit the eye and come out the mouth without going through the brain. It is the old joke of the definition of a college lecture—a place where the professor's notes are transferred to the students' notebooks without passing through the brain of either one. Speakers must constantly think about what they are saying and the meaning they want to convey. In addition, they must learn to watch the audience to determine whether they are getting the expected effect.

Robert Haakenson, PhD, is an outstanding speaker and a nationally recognized teacher of speaking. I have had the privilege of working as a co-director of one or two speaking workshops with him and have had the pleasure of reading a number of his brochures related to the field. One of them "How to Read a Speech" was published by Smith, Kline, and French Laboratories a few years back and contained some excellent advice, some of which is scattered throughout this book. In his brochure, he says "Reading a speech is death warmed over" (p. 1). He also comments very wisely, "Good reading conceals reading," and he adds, "Our reading will be impressive when our listeners have forgotten that it is reading" (p. 3).

Chapter 9

Use of Audiovisual Aids

INTRODUCTION

One of the greatest aids to teaching and lecturing has been the introduction and development of audiovisual aids. Slides, movies, tapes, and projectors have all added immeasurably to this second dimension of platform presentations. They have helped to make difficult and complicated subjects and material much more understandable.

However, as with all modern developments, there are dangers. The development of the automobile brought with it new problems, and the more sophisticated the auto became, the more complicated the problems. The same is true of television and airplanes. So it is with audiovisual aids for speeches. The development of these technical supports has brought widespread abuses, in part because of slavish dependency on them. These problems have reduced the potential enhancement value of audiovisual aids.

In today's lecture world, an overwhelming number of speakers believe that a lecture cannot be good unless slides are shown. (Some believe it is not a real lecture without slides.) That assumption has perverted what could be considered the actual aphorism: some, perhaps many, lecture presentations could be enhanced and improved with the addition of audiovisual aids. There once was a facetious expression that said, "An expert is a person from out of town with an attaché case." Today that has been changed to, "An expert is a person from out of town with a box of slides."

None of this is meant to discourage the use of slides. Instead, it is a commentary on what has happened when slides are used indiscriminately and without sufficient forethought—a situation that often occurs.

What is the ultimate audiovisual aid? Slides? Movies? No, it is a hands-on, three-dimensional demonstration of what the speaker is talking about. It could be an actual performance of a diagnostic technique, it could be simulation of cardiopulmonary resuscitation, or it could be an actual demonstration of a manipulation of the spine. All of these are excellent audiovisual aids, although not usually categorized as such. Let us look at how these ultimate forms would be used. Whatever the process, the speaker preparing to demonstrate it must use careful planning, focused attention to detail, and a perfected performance. No chances must be taken on the failure of the demonstration. If anything, more attention should be given to the demonstration than to the actual talk. The speaker knows that the actual demonstration will provide increased understanding to the audience. On the other hand, in today's world, it so often appears that medical slides—the most frequently used audiovisual aid—are indiscriminately or improperly used without regard to making them as good as the rest of the presentation.

The reason is simple. Good audiovisual presentations require extensive preparation, exquisite attention to detail, and knowledge of audiovisual techniques.

I hope to offer some insights to these approaches in this chapter. There is an additional dimension to audiovisual presentations that I shall avoid because it is not for the average speaker. I refer to the highly sophisticated, intricate presentations that take the form of unusual art work for slides, multiprojector slide shows, and multimedia presentations. These are in the realm of the professional audiovisual producer, and unless individual speakers have an unusual talent in this area, they should leave such approaches to the professional.

Therefore, I shall try to point out some of the common errors made in slide-show presentations and to offer some standard advice—the kind that helps most of us in the majority of our presentations. If this stimulates you to bigger and better audiovisual work, I would be very proud. If this information stimulates you to improve your everyday presentations, my goal will have been achieved.

MEDICAL AND TECHNICAL SLIDES

Medical slides, to be effective, must be easy to read, readily understood, clear and concise, and not shown too quickly or too slowly. Let us consider first the preparation of slides, dealing initially with printed material text on slides rather than pictures or diagrams.

Slides with Text

Before you can decide what to put on any slide, you must know in detail what you are going to talk about and what major points you are going to make. Using this topical outline for your presentation, you should then create for yourself a series of ideas that you want to present on slides to accompany your talk. Time spent on preproduction is extremely important and a requisite for real success.

Audiovisual professionals generally use a storyboard. This is a large board divided into blocks or on which are posted $3''$ x $5''$ cards, each containing a theme idea as well as the illustration or material that should go on a slide. These are placed in sequence, and then the sequence is manipulated to create the best story. Once this is done, the material for each slide can be developed and prepared.

Less complicated, perhaps, is to start by making a simple outline of your presentation. Then take an ordinary piece of paper and divide it in half down the center. Write the outline of your talk down the left-hand side of the page, and then place on the right-hand side of the page, corresponding to each major idea on the left, the material that you think will be most illustrative, for example, the wording of a slide or description of an illustration.

There are several pitfalls and errors that you can avoid by using this procedure:

1. You directly tie your slide to a specific topic or subject area.
2. It prevents you from putting massive amounts of material on a single slide.
3. You prevent copying your entire outline verbatim onto slides.

Too much material on a slide is one of the most counterproductive errors in slide presentations. Too many speakers put their full outlines on a slide and then lecture from the slides, thinking that this enhances their presentation. First, the viewers can review an entire slide in a few seconds and are well ahead of the speaker before the material can be discussed, thus confusing viewers rather than clarifying the presentation. If the only purpose of the slide is to provide an outline to guide the speaker in the talk, then the speaker is far better off giving the presentation without slides and speaking from a written outline. Why? To present slides, the room must be darkened; this diminishes the amount of personal interaction between speaker and audience and completely eliminates eye contact. This allows peoples' minds to drift off, and the speaker is more apt to lose the audience.

The real value of medical and technical slides is to project onto the screen material that will be more understandable to the eye than to the ear. This is why I have emphasized that slides should not be used as outline prompters for the speaker or to serve as notes for the lecture. This he or she can do just as well by keeping notes on hand when speaking. Text slides should be highlights projected to enhance and reinforce (by appealing to a second sense) the points being made by the speaker. Medical slides are really best when they show graphics, pictures, demonstrations, and other illustrative material.

Mary Evans, writing in the *British Medical Journal,* listed seven adjectives that describe good slides. She stated, "If more than two of the following adjectives do not apply to your slides scrap them and start again." The adjectives she presented were:

- appropriate
- accurate
- legible
- comprehensive
- well-executed
- interesting
- memorable

Succinctly, that is a great description of what slides ought to be.

Some Guidelines for Slides

Certain guidelines will assist your greatly in preparing better text slides for your talk:

1. Limit each slide to one main idea. By flashing a single idea and then explaining it, the speaker reinforces the point he or she is making. Multiple ideas may confuse the audience.
2. There should be a maximum of seven to nine lines on a slide, preferably six to seven. Authorities consider this a reasonable maximum, but I would advise using even fewer lines than this. The length of the line, too, should be brief, containing thirty-five to forty-nine characters in each line at the most, no more than six or seven words.
3. Prepare homemade slides with great care. If you use computer-generated slides or slides made by an art department, you have far fewer problems to worry about in this area.

However, many medical speakers do not have such facilities available to them and must make their own slides. If you do, remember that material for slides should never be typed on a manual typewriter. The electric typewriter gives you an even stroke so that the shading of the letters is uniform, provided the font faces are in good condition. Always use a mylar ribbon with the electric typewriter. Boldface type is the best and, if you have it available, a variable-spacing typewriter. Upper-case letters will improve the readability of your slides somewhat. If you have to underline items, use a steady India ink underlining; typewriter underlining tends to be uneven in shading and should not be used. Only perfect slides should be included in your talk; because of the nature of slides, corrections on a slide will be visible to the audience. If mistakes occur in the preparation, you should begin again. Before using your slides, proofread them very carefully. Lettering machines and computer software are available to improve even homemade slides. Whenever possible, use them. A template, which is an overlay or a pattern used as a guide, should be used so that you can determine whether your material will fit properly. Any typing should fit into the template ($2^1/_2''$ x $3^1/_4''$) (see Figure 9.1).

4. If you can read a slide with your naked eye, it probably can be read easily by your audience. If you cannot read it, the type is too small to be seen adequately by the audience.

5. Make your slides easier for the audience to read. Too often people experiment with fancy colors when simple colors will do. For best visualization, use a dark colored background; blue is probably better than black or white, and most people think the best combination is white letters on blue background; this is prepared by reversing your letters and ground. However, one color in each slide should be either black or white. Plain black typing on white back-

ground allows too much light and is more difficult to view; besides, it looks very amateurish.

6. Leave sufficient space between lines, to equal at least the height of a capital letter. This means the material should at least be double-spaced, allowing for greater readability of the slides.

7. Slides should be kept on the screen only for sufficient time for the audience to understand them. Slides need be left on the screen only for about ten to twelve seconds each. Up to thirty seconds should be the maximum time on the screen for any one slide, unless it is a chart or a drawing needing detailed explanation.

8. If you must discuss a single subject at length, use several simple slides rather than one complicated one.

9. Similarly, if your lecture contains progressive disclosure of a subject—for example, the Jones Criteria for the Diagnosis of Rheumatic Fever—it is better to have the first slide contain the first criterion for discussion, then the second slide should contain the first two criteria, with the second one accented or emphasized in the corresponding discussion. The remaining criteria should be presented similarly rather than putting all criteria on the screen at once (see Figure 9.2). If you plan to say a few words about each of the criteria, the description could be included on the individual slide which emphasizes that criterion and then eliminated in the next slide, which compiles all previous criteria (see Figure 9.3). This is a very simple device which requires no great creative ability to prepare but which multiplies the usefulness of the audiovisual portion of the presentation. Yet, it is rarely used except by very experienced presenters.

10. If you need to refer to the same slide—perhaps a basic outline of the subject you are talking about—at different times during your talk, duplicate that slide, and use one copy

for each instance in which you need it. This prevents you from trying to refer back to "slide one" or "that original outline which I showed you" or searching back through your presentation to find the slide. It keeps the material fresh in the minds of the viewers. It is extremely disruptive to an audience if slides are being flicked back and forth and also for the speaker because each time you must relocate where you left off. In addition, it is technically impractical for the projectionist to search for an old slide or to go back and make it reappear.

11. The speaker should explain the subject and not the words that appear on a slide, not simply read them to the audience. Remember that your listeners can also read and have already finished doing so before you even start to read aloud.

12. Run through your slides several times before the actual lecture so you can develop sequence and timing. Previewing your slides is as important as rehearsing your speech or rewriting a paper. Remember, you should be striving for a splendid talk.

13. Computer graphics and special software are making substantial inroads into platform presentations. The technology and mechanics are beyond the scope of this book, but a speaker should be aware of the benefits and limitations.

New computer software can help organize visual presentations and increase the viewers' ability to learn. Presentations may be transferred from computer-created and computer-stored information directly to the screen. When desired, 35 mm slides may also be made from the computer disk.

The market offers a number of software packages, such as Power Point, Astound, Applause, Hollywood, Harvard Graphics, Persuasion, and Presentations. Each speaker must explore these and determine which is best for him or her.

FIGURE 9.1. Template Setting Size for Typed Copy for Making Slides

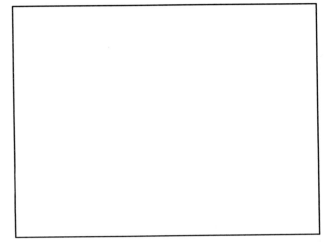

However, here is a caveat: all these technological advances are only *supplements* to your presentations. Your knowledge and your talk are the essential features. Don't get lost in *process* while diminishing the *substance*. Used judiciously, computerization (and all other aids) can improve, enhance, and clarify. Used indiscriminately, it can ruin your talk.

OVERHEAD PROJECTORS

As wth all other audiovisual aids, overhead projectors have certain advantages and disadvantages. One advantage is that overheads can be used in a lighted room while you face your audience throughout your presentation. Also, the cost of overhead transparencies is low, and they can be prepared in a short time.

However, if you use lettering for overhead projection, each letter should be at least one-quarter inch high; the disadvantage is that you cannot use ordinary typing, as many speakers try to do.

FIGURE 9.2. Illustrations Showing Progressive Disclosure with Emphasis on the Item Being Discussed

MAJOR MANIFESTATIONS
ACUTE RHEUMATIC FEVER

CARDITIS

Slide 1

MAJOR MANIFESTATIONS
ACUTE RHEUMATIC FEVER

CARDITIS

POLYARTHRITIS

Slide 2

MAJOR MANIFESTATIONS
ACUTE RHEUMATIC FEVER

CARDITIS

POLYARTHRITIS

CHOREA

Slide 3

MAJOR MANIFESTATIONS
ACUTE RHEUMATIC FEVER

CARDITIS

POLYARTHRITIS

CHOREA

ERYTHEMA MARGINATUM

Slide 4

MAJOR MANIFESTATIONS
ACUTE RHEUMATIC FEVER

CARDITIS

POLYARTHRITIS

CHOREA

ERTHEMA MARGINATUM

SUBCUTANEOUS NODULES

Slide 5

FIGURE 9.3. Examples of First Two Slides of a Similar Sequence Using Progressive Disclosure

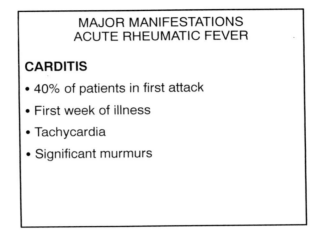

Slide 1

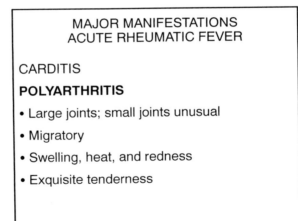

Slide 2

Note that each successive slide summarizes the major points covered and outlines in subheadings the salient features of the major manifestation under discussion.

My advice to you is this: do not use transparencies as a substitute for slides. If you are using transparencies only to show information or an illustration that can be put on a slide and projected, you will do much better with the slide. There are only three instances in which I would use an overhead projector:

1. It may be an alternative way (of about equal value) to show progressive divulgence of material instead of a projected slide. By putting a full page of material on the projector and then uncovering one line or two lines at a time to show progression, you will have a valuable teaching tool. However, this can be done just as well with regular projection slides (but at a greater cost).

2. Second, there is the occasional time when you want to show an audience that you could talk about a multitude of items. For example, if you wanted to impress your audience with the number of causes of fever that exist, you might briefly present a transparency with two columns listing diseases that cause fever. However, if the rest of your presentation is slides, do not use a transparency; put it on a slide or slides. If you are teaching with transparencies, then it is satisfactory to make this use of it.

3. Third, and the most important use of all, is when you plan to use transparencies to teach by modifying what is printed on them. For example, in conducting writing seminars, I put a page or two of a manuscript on transparencies. Then, using a china marking crayon, I edit the transparency with the audience while they watch the transformation from an unedited script to an edited script. This working use of the transparency is by far its greatest value.

CHALK TALKS

Chalk talks are simple presentations in which the speaker gives the talk and writes significant explanatory items or illustrations on a blackboard or whiteboard. The major advantage is that, properly presented, the audio (speech) blends fully with the visual (the chalkboard) to form an integrated talk. These talks tend to be more understandable and are easier to give; they require no preliminary mechanical preparation (such as slides or transparencies). The only limitation seems to be that the speaker's back is to the audience a portion of the time, but with experience using this type of presentation, this becomes a minimal handicap.

Chalk talks are good for smaller groups, perhaps twenty-five to fifty people. Beyond this size, it is difficult to write large enough and clearly enough on a blackboard or whiteboard for an audience to see.

VIDEOTAPES

A word should be said about the use of videotapes. First, they should be carefully selected and screened. They should be completely applicable if you are going to show the entire tape, and they should not be too long, unless the video is the main part of the presentation. Arrangements should be made in advance so that the start and end of the tape or of the section you are showing flows in smoothly with the talk so that everything comes off without a hitch (preferably someone should be there to help you). Be sure that the video player is the same size as the tape you plan to use.

Videotapes have a distinct advantage in teaching (and sometimes in talks): you can stop the tape and comment on it or even go back and replay the last part, after your commentary, so the audience can see what you are talking about. You can stop the film and actually point to specific or important parts. There is great flexibility in the use of videotapes.

In this chapter, I have attempted to develop a primer on the use of medical slides, not present an intensive course in audiovisual aids. Use of these suggestions will greatly improve any speaker's slides. For those who already use these recommendations, and for those who would like to go deeper into the technical aspects of medical slides, there is an abundant supply of books and other information. Every library has some material and much can be found at colleges and universities where there is a school of communication. One of the most complete and helpful sources is Kodak, and lists of their available information and brochures may be obtained from the Motion Picture and Audiovisual Markets Division, Rochester, New York 14650.

Chapter 10

Introductions

I attended a convention not long ago at which the moderator introduced almost every speaker with the same trite line: "The next speaker is Dr. Smith." That constituted the entire introduction. No first names. No titles. No topics. Many members of the organization were embarrassed because among the speakers were several of national prominence.

This not-so-rare occurrence highlights the very reason for introductions: a speaker worth having in a program deserves an appropriate introduction. Otherwise, name, title, and topic could appear on a written program, and each speaker would automatically follow the previous speaker without any introductions. Even if this information is printed on the program, it is not sufficient reason to shortchange the speaker or the audience by using a weak or absent introduction.

Introductions come in a variety of styles and qualities, anywhere from brilliant to mundane to horrible. Every professional who may be called upon to introduce colleagues or visiting guests should have a reasonable concept of what is expected of an introduction and should take this assignment as seriously as he or she takes an actual speaking assignment. Introductions require preparation and attention to detail. Organizations should choose their introducers as carefully as they select their speakers; these positions should not be routinely assigned to a certain officer, such as the vice president.

First, if the introducer (chairperson or moderator) is the first on the program to speak, it becomes his duty to greet the audience, welcome them, and say a word or two about the program. More about this appears in Chapter 11, "Being a Program Moderator." Introductions should include the speaker's full name, along with an important title or affiliation.

Should the speaker be introduced as Dr. Samuel Jones or as Samuel Jones, PhD—or DO or MD or DDS? That depends on the program and on the length and content of the introduction that is planned. If introductions are to be short, giving the speaker's degree is a concise way to describe his or her background. If on the other hand, you are planning to tell where the speaker graduated from, trained, or interned or intend to tell the audience that the speaker is Chairperson of the Department of Anesthesiology at Massachusetts General Hospital, giving a degree may be unnecessary. If this information appears in the printed program, it is probably unnecessary to state the degree—the title doctor will suffice. The program, too, helps determine whether to use the speaker's degree. For example, at a dental society meeting with almost all dentist speakers, the degree is needed only for those who are not dentists.

All this applies if a printed program is available and distributed at the meeting; if it has been mailed only, do not assume that anyone has read it. Give speakers their due, as if the audience does not know them.

How much should be told about the speaker? Again, this depends on the time available for introductions. There should be some correlation between the expected length of the speech and the length of the introduction. If the speech is to be ten minutes long, the introduction should not be five minutes—it probably should be a minute or less. On the other hand, a lecture of forty-five or sixty minutes deserves a longer introduction, but not a lot longer.

Sometimes brevity is the best introduction. Probably the briefest, best, and most effective introduction we know is the universally used "Ladies and gentlemen, the President of the United

States." Since most of us never come anywhere near introducing a personality of that magnitude, it is probably important that more be included.

Most of us, as introducers, depend on the curriculum vitae of the speaker as a base for our information. However, if you know interesting personal things about the speaker (providing they do not embarrass the speaker), including them will make your introduction much more powerful and listenable. Compare the two introductions below:

1. Ladies and gentlemen, our speaker tonight is a nationally known internist, whose work in endocrinology has made his name a household word. He comes to us from Stanford University where he is Professor of Medicine. Ladies and gentlemen, Dr. Charles Smith.
2. We have a real treat and pleasure today. Our speaker, Dr. Charles Smith, is not only nationally known as an endocrinologist and a member of the faculty at Stanford University, but he is more important to us: he is responsible for training our own endocrinologist, Bill White, and is a second cousin to George Apple, our cardiologist. So he comes not only as an authority and as a distinguished guest, but almost as a member of the family. Ladies and gentlemen, Dr. Charles Smith.

Unfortunately, many introducers misuse the curriculum vitae (CV) of the speaker, by committing one of the two common errors. The worst introductions occur when the introducer takes the CV directly to the podium and leafs through it, searching for accomplishments and titles as he introduces the speaker. Most of these introducers create the impression of never having reviewed the CV in advance. The introducer may have marked the titles he or she wants to read but nevertheless turns six or eight pages during the introduction. This is quite disconcerting to the audience; It makes them think the introducer doesn't know anything about the speaker. How much simpler it is to copy those titles onto a piece of paper and use that as a reference to introduce the speaker. As I have said before, preparation is a significant part of introductions.

However, using five or six titles may lead to the other error, although it is less offensive: The introducer reads the CV verbatim to the audience. CVs were not meant to be *read* to audiences. They are a listing of a person's accomplishments for academic or other purposes. An introduction, however, should be a story about the person. It is meant to acquaint your audience with the person whose accomplishments, it might be assumed, only you know in detail at the moment. Woven into it should be a number of accomplishments so that when you are finished the audience has a brief but clear and concise picture of who and what the speaker is.

The most perfect example of such an ideal introduction is the presentation of a distinguished person for an honorary degree or a special award. The presenter never reads a curriculum vitae or lists the titles and accomplishments, but rather weaves a story that gives the audience a very clear and compact picture—who this person is, including background and experience, and the reason for honoring him or her.

This is an actual example (name changed) of a presentation of an award during a graduation ceremony:

I have the privilege of presenting Dr. Marcus Morgan to receive our Distinguished Service Award.

After graduation from medical school, Dr. Morgan moved to Florida and established a successful general practice. He was highly respected by patients and peers alike. Later he turned his talents toward medical education.

Marc is a medical educator in the fullest sense of the word. He has degrees in osteopathic medicine and in educational administration. As Director of Medical Education in two osteopathic hospitals, he has created educational programs for house staff, for hospitals, and for professional associations for many years.

An outstanding member of the Academy of Osteopathic Directors of Medical Education, he is a Fellow of that organization and has served as its president. Recently the governor appointed him to membership in the prestigious Community Hospital Education Council, the first osteopathic physician ever named to this board.

There is a wonderful song from *Oklahoma* titled, "I'm Just a Girl Who Can't Say No." Dr. Morgan is just a guy who won't say no. In the nine years we have been in existence, he has never declined any task we presented to him.

He served on the Dean's Advisory Council on Curriculum even before the first class entered. He is a key member of our Admissions Committee and of the important Curriculum Committee. At his two hospitals, he supervises the training of our students on clinical rotations with singular dedication. In a myriad of things which defy categorization, Marcus Morgan responded every time we asked him. And he responded willingly, diligently, and successfully.

Marcus Morgan is truly our man who won't say no and I am delighted to present him to receive this Distinguished Service Award.

This presentation is editorialized, with personal comments, and contains words of praise. It is literally a sales pitch; it should make the audience anxious to hear the speaker—that's what makes it a fine introduction.

Unimportant items, or relatively unimportant items, should be left out of introductions. If the speaker has been elected president of an organization, for example, the American Public Health Association, it is only necessary to make that single statement; the presumption would be that he or she served in a number of committee appointments, other offices, and other positions in that organization before becoming President of APHA. Therefore, it is not necessary, in addition to saying he or she is President, to point out that the individual served as Chairperson of the Membership Committee or Chairperson of the Child Health Section prior to becoming President.

Another common error made is for an introducer to say "Dr. Green has such a voluminous CV that I will not attempt to read it to you, so here he is," or some words to that effect. This not only eliminates the opportunity to say something nice about this speaker but is an insult to him. You can assume that a speaker invited to an important function has accumulated a reasonable curriculum vitae, and the actual size of it does not make a huge difference. In fact, an introduction that says, "Ronald Reagan served as Governor of the State of California, his first elective office, and is now President of the United States," probably says much more than listing all of the committee appointments that some of us have filled in a lifetime.

Most appropriate in this regard is the famous story of the legendary Minnie Guggenheim, who sponsored and hosted the Lewisohn Stadium Concerts in New York for many years. One evening, Mrs. Guggenheim, in trying to heap exceptional praise on the world-famous violinist Isaac Stern, is reported to have said "Would you believe that Isaac Stern's 'Who's Who' is almost seven inches long?" Although this has gone down as one of the unforgettable introductions of all time, she did not mean to be funny—she meant to be complimentary. Other introducers have trapped themselves into similar binds by lack of preparation and forethought.

One gaffe that is not uncommon is the failure to pronounce a speaker's name or the name of one of his or her organizations correctly. Once again, this generally indicates lack of preparation, or it may be taken by the audience as indifference, or even as insulting. To mispronounce "osteopathic" or "podiatric," for example, or the name of the speaker's hometown, is an affront to the listeners and to the speaker. It embarrasses a speaker with a difficult or foreign name when you mispronounce it, or worse, stammer over it. All of us are obligated to prepare our introductions carefully and to learn to pronounce any difficult names, without embarrassment to the speaker, the audience, or ourselves.

Try to avoid trite, overused expressions, such as, "It is my pleasure to introduce . . ." or "It is a pleasure and a privilege . . ." Just converting these two clichés from passive to active voice (even if that's all you do) makes a great improvement. It is much better to say "I am pleased (honored, overjoyed) to introduce . . .". Just a little bit of interest in the task, a little concern for the speaker, and a lot of concern for the audience will enable almost every introducer to create something a bit more listenable. Every introduction does not have to be ingenious and brilliant, but all can avoid being dull and repetitious.

Having said all this about introductions, the most important qualities of an introduction—any introduction, long, short, detailed, sketchy, friend, stranger—are enthusiasm, warmth, and an apparent interest in the speaker and his or her topic. The introducer must appear (and act) enthusiastic about the program and the topic and especially the speaker. He or she must be warm and friendly, and the audience must feel that the introducer himself or herself can hardly wait to hear what the speaker has to say.

In a community which will be nameless, at an annual lecture series which will also be nameless, a brilliant chairman introduced each evening's guest. His presentation followed all the "rules" I have cited, and after five minutes, you felt you knew the speaker well and wanted strongly to hear the speech. But then—every time—this introducer proceeded (as a way of introducing the speaker's topic) to discuss in detail the subject of the speaker's talk. Endlessly. Boringly. At the cost of almost destroying the night for each speaker. Lesson to be learned: even if you do it right, know when to stop. You are introducing the speaker, not giving the speech.

A WORD ABOUT CLOSINGS

Perhaps this chapter could have been called "Introductions and Closings," but since the preponderance of material is on introductions, I did not do so.

In most instances, the person who introduces the speaker also closes the meeting or concludes the program. The order in which the introducer concludes the program has no special meaning, but it should make sense to the audience. Several items should be included in this conclusion:

- Commentary on the subject matter of the presentation (it need not be discussed in detail or rehashed, but some sort of indication of its importance should be made)
- Acknowledgement of the importance of the talk and the speaker to the program being presented
- Thanks to the speaker
- Praise for the job he or she has done

In most instances, these points can be covered rather briefly, while you still pay sufficient respect to the speaker and his or her talk. In unusual situations, the introducer may want to make these remarks a bit more elaborate, but there is very rarely the need for making prolonged remarks at this point, possibly upstaging the guest speaker. When these points have been covered, the introducer then either introduces the next speaker or indicates that the meeting has come to a close.

Chapter 11

Being a Program Moderator

If you have been asked to be a moderator of a panel discussion or a symposium and you are delighted, do you feel that you will have very little work to do? Wrong. Presiding over one of these functions is as serious a matter as giving a speech and, in some ways, is more taxing. As with any professional talk, it requires good preparation, high concentration, and excellent platform skills.

First of all, "panel discussion" and "symposium" are often used interchangeably, and very often only the program chairperson knows what he or she means when the program is set up. Therefore, such program events may vary from situation to situation, and there are many (and conflicting) definitions of these two terms.

For the purposes of discussion here, I have provided definitions that will distinguish these two types of programs. As we shall use the terms in this chapter, a symposium is a program unit, generally devoted to one topic or one aspect of a topic, in which there are several participants. The participants deliver individual talks, each on a different aspect of the symposium topic. They are individually introduced by the moderator as each one reaches his or her turn to talk. Following this, there may or may not be a question-and-answer period; symposium does not necessarily imply the presence or absence of a questioning period.

By panel discussion, I mean an interactive program unit, with participation by several different persons, in which aspects of a specific topic may be discussed or in which each speaker discusses views and opinions on the same topic. It is characterized by an interchange of opinion and ideas rather than single individual talks. This definition does not preclude each speaker giving an initial presentation of a few minutes to establish for the audience a position or a few ideas. Some panel discussions allow each speaker a few moments to introduce views on a subject and then all of the remainder of the time is spent in allowing the panel members to discuss their own ideas or give their comments on other speakers' presentations. In either case, the discussion here is applicable.

A Word About the Moderator

Although more will be said about this most important person, let me point out up front that the success or failure of such panels depends a great deal on the moderator. This person's interest, knowledge of the subject, appreciation of the personalities of the panel members, and interplay with the audience can make a silk purse out of a sow's ear—or a sow's ear out of a silk purse.

As you read the duties and attributes of the moderator in the following discussions, keep in mind how important that role is.

SYMPOSIA

If the moderator is not introduced by a program chairperson or an officer of the group, it is the moderator's duty to introduce himself or herself, to explain the purpose of the symposium, to introduce the participants, and to introduce the topic. When a moderator is introduced by another person, he or she must then modify these duties appropriately so that there is no repetition for the audience. There are program chairpersons who may usurp the prerogative of the symposium moderator and introduce all of the participants. In this case, the moderator simply eliminates this particular step.

Let us hypothesize a symposium in which the moderator has not been introduced. The moderator moves to the podium and begins:

> Good morning, fellow members of the American Cardiology Guild. Since your program called for a symposium on "The Cholesterol Factors in Heart Disease" at 10:00 a.m., and since it is now 10:00 a.m., we must both make some assumptions. I must assume that you are present to hear this symposium, and you must assume that our distinguished speakers are ready to participate in that symposium.
>
> My name is Bill Nottingham. I am today's moderator, and when I am not conducting symposia, I am a professor of cardiology at Standard College of Medicine.

At this point, it is appropriate for the moderator to introduce the panel members. The length and detail of these introductions depends on the amount of biography included in the printed program, on what has been said about them previously, on whether they have been introduced before during the course of the program, and on the length of the symposium. The first three factors provide obvious leads for the moderator.

The length of introduction should bear a relationship to the total length of the program. These guidelines apply for any introduction of a speaker. For a thirty-minute symposium (which would be very short), the introduction of all the participants (if they are the first introductions) should not use up more than a couple of minutes of the symposium time. For example:

> With me on the platform this morning are three distinguished cardiologists: Dr. Samuel Goodman, Professor of Medicine at Northeastern Medical School, who has written extensively on topics relating to high density lipoproteins; Dr. Alexandra Rootin, Associate Professor of Cardiology at Springfield University School of Medicine, who has an extensive re-

search background in the relationship between cholesterol and triglycerides; and Dr. Phillip Mc Connell, a PhD in Biochemistry at New York's Brookline Hospital.

Having introduced the symposium as well as the participants, it is now the moderator's duty to give the audience a brief insight into the problem being discussed. Again, the length of introduction depends on the length of the program time. Let us continue our example of a brief symposium:

Before I turn the panel loose, it would be wise to set the stage for our discussions. As all of you know, cholesterol and other lipoproteins have been indicted as causes of coronary occlusion. Among the related compounds that have been studied as risk factors is triglyceride and other related lipoproteins. There has been much new material from laboratories, from biochemical research, and from clinical experts, to aid those of us who treat such patients. However, enough is still unknown that it can lead to the opportunity, such as today, to discuss the disparate opinions. I will ask Dr. Goodman to begin the symposium by presenting a brief view of his opinions on this important topic.

As each speaker finishes his or her introductory presentation, the moderator briefly presents the next speaker in turn.

When all of the speakers have been introduced and have given their initial presentations, the work of the moderator really begins. Two general avenues are open: first, the moderator can ask whether any of the panel members have questions of other panel members or wish to comment on previous statements; second, the moderator can raise one or several pertinent questions of his or her own, based on the discussions in the symposium thus far. Then, the moderator can ask other participants to comment. The questions may have been prepared in advance, or they may arise as the discussions proceed. Both methods are meant to stimulate thinking and audience participation.

From this point on, the moderator is like the gatekeeper at a bullfight—not participating but opening the gate whenever necessary to "let a little bull out at a time." His or her job is to keep the discussion moving (and sometimes this means raising questions or making statements to move the discussion along). It is the moderator's duty to do either of these whenever there is a lull in the discussion or when no questions are forthcoming from the audience. The moderator must see that all the panel members participate and that no one or two "hog" the discussion, and he or she must draw out the reticent members of the panel. It is the moderator's ability in professional speaking and skill in interpersonal relationships that will play the biggest role in ensuring the success of the symposium.

One or two minutes before the end of the time allotted for the symposium, the moderator must halt the discussions (it is his or her fault if the symposium goes overtime!) and summarize, in a matter of a few sentences, the consensus of the symposium and the remaining differences of opinion. Finally, the moderator turns to the speakers and thanks them individually by name.

The closing of a symposium calls for as much attention as the closing of a speech. Trail-offs (described earlier), trite closings, and indefinite endings have no place. A strong closing remark, preferably tied into the topic, speakers, organization, or symposium would be most appropriate. For example, if the symposium produced a great deal of debate and difference of opinion, an appropriate closing might be:

This morning certainly has not proved to be a morning of agreement. Here you have heard a wide divergence of opinion, all of it authoritative. We all understand how important the lipoproteins and triglycerides are in the cholesterol problem, and we hope that this exciting discussion has helped you reach your own conclusions or stimulated you to follow the subject more intensively.

This ending does not drop off or fizzle out. It concludes with a positive statement and ends with strength.

Please note a special prejudice of mine. I dislike the use of hackneyed expressions in any speaking situation. Although the examples I have given are just examples, you should note that I have not resorted to such expressions as "Thank you for listening," "It is my privilege to present _____ ," or any others. With a little thought, most speakers can be clever and innovative, even on a small scale—at least they can avoid being trite.

There is a postscript for moderators. When a symposium has ended, it is polite for the moderator to shake hands with all the participants and to thank them for their part in making the symposium so successful. If the moderator has also been responsible for choosing and inviting the participants, he or she should send a note of thanks to each speaker as soon as possible after the conclusion of the symposium.

PANEL DISCUSSIONS

Most of what has been said about symposia can also be applied to panel discussions. In a panel discussion, the moderator has a choice of introducing all the speakers at the beginning of the program, with appropriate biographical material (and subsequently presenting each one in turn by name only), or introducing each speaker as he or she is about to talk. Both approaches have their values and both have their advocates. It is best for the moderator to pick the one with which he or she is most comfortable. All of the remaining parameters are the same.

Between presentations of the speakers, the moderator, who should have real knowledge of the subject, should comment very briefly about the previous speaker's remarks and lead into the next speaker's presentation. This interval between speakers, filled by the moderator's comments, actually serves a couple of purposes: it provides a segue from one talk to another, and serves as an opportunity for members of the audience to relax a bit, stretch, make a comment to a neighbor, or make themselves more comfortable in their seats.

During the symposium, when panelists are speaking, it is the responsibility of the moderator to be (or at least appear to be) totally interested in what is going on. He or she must not yield to distractions (because the moderator does not want the audience to be distracted), and he or she must never appear bored or annoyed, no matter how much he or she knows about the subject.

Always remember, the moderator is not the star of a panel discussion, but rather the catalyst that makes the stars shine, and in this respect, is a key element in the symposium's success.

QUESTIONS AND ANSWERS

The question-and-answer period can be the icing on the cake that makes the symposium successful, or it can be the drain down which the symposium flushes itself.

The first problem encountered in asking for questions is that in a majority of situations there is reluctance on the part of members of the audience to be the first questioner.

Exhortations of the moderator, or pleading with the audience, are rather useless and embarrassing. The moderator should always be prepared to make a thought-provoking statement or summary to the audience as he or she opens the questioning period. This is meant to give members of the audience either additional time to crystallize their questions or to raise their courage. (Yes, even asking questions at a meeting takes some of the same courage as needed in making a speech.)

If no one in the audience asks a question and if the moderator's initial statement does not stimulate any questions, the moderator should ask a direct question of one of the speakers. In fact, it is wise for the moderator to have prepared at least one question in advance for each speaker and then use these questions to stimulate the audience or to fill in lulls.

The same parameters for questions and answers in a symposium or panel are applicable to all situations in which Q and A is used.

Chapter 12

Humor in Professional Speaking

Humor is that very delicate ingredient which adds to a talk as seasoning adds to a sauce. It is not a primary factor, except in talks by humorists, but it adds spice and zest to almost all presentations. It cannot make a poor talk good; it cannot make a dull talk interesting, but it can improve most speeches.

Not everyone can use humor, and not everyone can be successful with the same type of humor. Not everyone should try. Some humor should be attempted in a speech, and most speakers should learn to do what they can with humor to enliven their presentations. However, if you find yourself unsuccessful in using humor, eliminate it.

Where are the best places to introduce humor? Almost any place in the talk where it is appropriate would be satisfactory. The first logical place that one may add humor is in response to an introduction. The second would be as an icebreaker for the talk. Third, during the talk, the speaker may want to add something humorous as relief from a long stretch of serious discussion, as a change of pace, or as an interesting illustration. Finally, it is always appropriate in a summary of the talk or as the haymaker in the finale. It is quite effective when used as a "walk-off," that is, when the very final thing the speaker does is to deliver the punch line of a funny story (which has met the necessary tests of being illustrative, appropriate, and in good taste) and leave the platform.

OPENING HUMOR

One of my favorite stories for use as an opening or icebreaker is the chauffeur joke in Chapter 6. It has never failed to get a hearty laugh and to put the audience in a good mood for the rest of my remarks.

There have been occasions when I have been invited back to speak to a group a second or third time. Among my favorite icebreakers for these occasions are the following:

> Since this is the second time I have been invited here, I worried the entire time while driving here, fearful that you might feel like the second grade teacher in one of our neighboring schools. When she walked into her class one day, she noticed as she passed the cloakroom that the middle of the floor was wet. Holding her anger, she stood before the class and said, "Children, as I passed the cloakroom I noticed a puddle in the middle of the floor. We are all going to put our heads down on our desks, and I want the person responsible for that puddle to go back and do the proper thing. Now all of you put your heads down on the desks." There was silence, then the patter of little feet, then silence again, then the patter of little feet. At this point the teacher was proud of the way she handled the problem and said, "Children, you may now raise your heads." She walked over to the cloakroom and there on the floor was a second puddle, and next to it a note with a childish scawl, "The Phantom strikes again!" I certainly hope you won't regard me as The Phantom today.

Or as an icebreaker immediately following a particularly flowery introduction:

> (In a very serious tone) At this point, I feel compelled to invoke what has come to be known as the Speaker's Prayer: Dear Lord, please forgive the chairman for his exaggerated

remarks about me. And dear Lord, please forgive me for believing them.

In other instances, I have used a similar short, punchy icebreaker:

Mr. Chairman I wish my mother and father could be here tonight to hear that beautiful introduction. My father would have been so proud . . . and my mother would have believed every word of it!

Please note that in every one of these instances, I actually started speaking with the first word of each example as the first word of my talk—nothing else before it. From these introductions, I then made a transition into another portion of my opening or directly into my talk.

CLOSING HUMOR

Humor as a closing for a talk, if the humor is appropriate and effective, can add an excellent note to your speech. I referred previously to the "walk-off." A favorite "walk-off" story is one that I often used when I lectured on childhood behavior, child psychology, or similar subjects. After discussing in depth a number of serious points (interlaced with humor) about the behavior of children, I concluded with:

I still remember one of my patients who read a good bit of pop psychology and thought she knew all about handling children. When her five-year-old got out of hand one day and nothing the mother said or did controlled her, the mother screamed, "You get in that closet and you stay there until I tell you to come out." The weeping five-year-old went into the closet. All was silent. Five minutes. Silence. Ten minutes. Silence. The mother, exhausting all her "scientific knowledge" and in total frustration, tore open the door, looked down at the sobbing little girl and said, "What are you doing in there?" The little girl looked up tearfully and sobbed, "I'm thpittin' on your dreth . . . and I'm thpittin' on your thatin thlippers . . . " Mother said, "And what else?" "And I'm waiting for more thpitt."

Another piece of humor that I have frequently used, which is not a walk-off but provides a strong closing, is this one:

A few weeks ago, I was returning from a trip to Texas. I sat down in my usual seat on the aisle, and as I did so, I noticed a very attractive young lady entering the plane. I watched her as she found her place—the window seat across the aisle from me. At that point I was aware of a "typical" Texan entering. Tall, boots, and a ten-gallon Stetson. He sat down in the aisle seat just across from me. But he too saw this attractive young lady. He turned to her and smiled and said, "Good mornin', ma'am." The young lady abruptly turned her head and looked out the window, totally ignoring him. He waited a few moments and tried again, "Nice morning, isn't it, Ma'am?" Again she rudely turned away and looked out the window. The plane took off, and as we reached cruising altitude, he tried once more, "You travelin' on business or pleasure, Ma'am?" For the third time, he received the same icy rejection. This was enough even for a Texan, so he slumped his 6'4" frame down into the seat, pushed his Stetson forward over his face, and promptly fell asleep. When the plane arrived and taxied to the gate, he awoke, pulled himself up to his full height, and once more smiled at the young lady. "Ma'am," he said, "our conversation wasn't very much but I shore enjoyed sleeping with ya." Now, I don't know how many of you were sleeping during my talk but I "shore enjoyed being with ya."

No matter what the humor, it should always tie into the talk that is being given, or it should be made to tie in. True, those tie-ins may have to be tenous at times if the connection is not obvious, but the speaker must attempt to make the humor sound appropriate.

DIALECT STORIES

The humor chosen by the speaker should be what he or she can use with comfort. For example, dialect stories, although frowned upon in most instances, may be appropriate under certain circumstances, but only if the dialect portion is essential to the humor of the story and is in no way pejorative. There are some great speakers who are capable of using dialect stories that apply to their own backgrounds. A good Irish speaker, for example, can get away with almost any kind of Irish brogue story, if it is appropriate to the talk.

However, dialect stories are fraught with danger: people are easily offended by them. My advice: leave them alone unless you have extensive experience in telling them and the sophistication to read your audiences' potential reactions. Experts can use dialect stories effectively; the late Myron Cohen, one of America's best storytellers, could do any of several dialects and never offend.

If used, the dialect must be an integral part of the joke or connect with the talk. Never make a story black, Jewish, Polish, or any other ethnic group just for the sake of using it; it must be appropriate.

The dialect itself must be true and well-done. It must not be forced or faked or stereotyped. If you can't mimic a particular dialect, do not use it; it will be intrinsically insulting.

The dialect must not be offensive in any way. Be certain not to use a dialect joke that may seem appropriate to the occasion, but that could be insulting or demeaning to members of your audience.

All of this applies to ethnic humor also. And to sexist humor.

"OFF-COLOR" STORIES

"Off-color" stories are almost always inappropriate, but the interpretation of what is off-color and what is not varies with the speaker and the audience. Truly "blue" material should never be used in a professional talk, but sometimes slightly off-color but appropriate humor may fit a particular situation. The story of the Texan, found a few pages back, is one of these.

Never use off-color stories if a "clean" story will do. Never use an off-color story to "impress," "shock," or "defy" your audience. But, under any circumstances, you must feel comfortable telling the story or you should not use it. When in doubt, the answer is "No." It is far better to eliminate humor than to be or appear to be uncomfortable with what you are doing. Just because the hospital administrator laughed at it in the lobby, just because the doctors in the dressing room convulsed, and just because your friends giggled in the parking lot does not justify using that same material from the public platform.

The second criterion for choosing humor is what the audience will accept. You owe your audience the courtesy of total consideration. For example, there is a great deal of difference between speaking before a young college-age group (especially today) and a staid, elderly women's group. Also, the age of the speaker must be taken into consideration. Before you plan humor, examine whether your audience will accept something slightly off-color or ethnic. Who are they? What are their feelings? What mores do they have? Most important of all, as I've said before, is appropriateness to the occasion, and this depends on both the audience and the situation. Young ribald comedians often lace their routines with four-letter words when appearing before college audiences; a sixty-year old comedian (or speaker) would certainly be out of place doing the same thing.

Reading this may make you think I am a straightlaced prude and that I am recommending that you be the same. Rubbish. I have told my share of ethnic, dialect, and off-color stories—they can be effective audience winners. However, I hope that I have always used discretion and good judgment in using them. I must relate two stories as cautionary examples:

> I attended a banquet honoring some students and there were a number of talks. Toward the end of the dinner, a class representative was called upon to respond on behalf of the students. He went to the microphone and made a fairly appropriate tie-in by saying, "A funny thing happened to me in the hotel elevator this afternoon." He then proceeded to tell a dirty story (not just off-color) whose punch line contained a bleep word for which he had the sense to provide a substitute. The oncoming punch line was obvious from the context of the story, and when the audience realized what it would be, they literally gasped. When he finished, even though there was some laughter, many people in the audience were aghast that he had not used better judgment. Good judgment is the key to selecting stories.

> A large nightclub in Philadelphia used to be open on Thanksgiving afternoon for family dinners. They were always packed with a large number of children as well as the adults. On one occasion, one of the world's best storytellers was the star of the show. This was a man who had, with good judgment, told stories for presidents, royalty, and everyone else. On this occasion, in the midst of a routine, he apparently thought of another story. However, the punch line contained one locker-room word, and that word was the crux of the joke. When he finished, there was deadly silence in the audience. There was not one titter, not one giggle, not one laugh. Being a seasoned

performer, he immediately realized his gross error; he apologized, and he continued to apologize throughout the remainder of his act. Not only did his performance that day fail because of lack of judgment, but his reputation sank to the bottom in the minds of almost every person in that nightclub. Notice that even professionals make mistakes, so certainly those of us who only dabble in storytelling should exercise extra care and judgment.

HOW TO USE HUMOR

There are many "don'ts" for the delivery of humor for the speaker who is inexperienced in its use. Think seriously about the following:

- Don't read a joke. Reading a joke makes it dull and boring. If you cannot tell a story from memory, it is not worth telling, and it will fail because it has been read. Every joke that is told should be practiced very carefully; you should never tell a story for the first time when giving your talk. You must practice!
- Don't telegraph your joke. Telegraphing is giving clues, consciously or unconsciously, that you are about to tell a joke. That includes saying, "This reminds me of a story," or any similar trite introduction. Tie your joke into your speech material and try to "segue" it. "Segue" is a term generally used in broadcasting to describe two disparate things that are tied together with a smooth transition. Segueing humor is very appropriate and should be practiced by every speaker.
- Don't tell impersonal stories if you can avoid it. Don't say, "This man walked into a store" or "A woman purchased a hat." Always try to personalize a story by attributing it to yourself, someone in the audience (without being insulting), or someone that the audience recognizes. Make it specific

and refer to people by name whenever possible. However, be certain that you are insulting no one. It is far better, if possible, to tell the joke "on yourself."

- Don't make your stories long. Keep them as short as possible because if you are a poor storyteller you will bore your audience with a long story. If they have heard the story before, you will be wasting their time. Notice sometime that professionals (comedians for example), when telling a long story, intersperse funny lines to keep the audience's interest until they reach the big punch line. The beginning speaker might learn to try one-liners as a start.
- Don't apologize for your humor. It is not a good idea to apologize for your story by making such comments as, "I'm not a very good storyteller, but . . . " or "Maybe you heard this story but anyhow . . . " This speaker is telling the audience to expect a poor performance. It is better, if these statements are true, not to tell the story at all or even not to use humor.
- Don't make yourself a hero unless it is germane to the talk. It is far more humorous when the speaker makes himself or herself the butt of a joke. This is particularly true following introductions, especially if an introduction is extremely flowery. A good joke about yourself, which implies modesty or less achievement or ability than the introducer described, would be appropriate. Most experienced speakers have prepared acceptances for introductions (some humorous, some not), and they use them depending on the introduction. You might look back at the earlier ones in this chapter.

You have heard speakers make comments such as, "It's true, that's just the way I wrote it" or "Your introduction was so great I can hardly wait to hear my speech." These are trite examples that you should not use because they have been overworked and are no longer funny. However, they do illustrate prepared replies to fancy introductions. Even though I do not care for lines such as these, I used one on a recent occasion (because I had a reason). I was introduced by a noted pharmacist with a very flowery presentation. On arising, I said, "Everything he said is true. It's exactly the way I wrote it for him." (Unexpectedly, the audience laughed considerably—which again proves the point that a joke is old only if you've heard it before.) At this point, I added my spontaneous comment, which tied into my opening joke and matched the occasion, "And that's the first time in ages a pharmacist has been able to read a physician's handwriting so easily." The laughter was considerable, and I was on my way.

• Don't berate the audience for not laughing. Every storyteller and every speaker has had jokes fall flat. Sometimes you think that the joke you are telling is the funniest one you have ever heard in your life. Perhaps even several audiences have roared with laughter at it, but you tell it to another audience, and there is a dull thud. Jokes have a way of affecting different audiences differently, and since you do not feel exactly the same every time you speak, you may even unconsciously tell it differently on different occasions.

Situations and circumstances change, and the audience reaction to what you say may change. There is a story (probably apocryphal) about two actors discussing a play in which they were performing. "Did you notice the great laugh I got in the second act when I almost dropped the champagne glass?" said one. "You?" replied the other. "That's the same time that I'm making faces in the mirror." After considerable debate, they decided to test it out. That night, the first actor didn't touch the champagne glass. No laughter. "See, I told you," said the second actor. Then they tried the reverse—play with the champagne glass but no faces in the mirror. No laughter. The answer was obvious to them—the combination elicited the laughter. That night, they went back to the original. BUT NO LAUGHTER. The "chemistry" was gone; something they had been doing subconsciously—the combination—brought forth laughter, but they were unaware of what they did. Never again in the run of the play did that scene get a laugh. So don't worry about different reactions to your humor from different audiences.

You must remember that all jokes are not guffaws. Some of them just elicit a snicker or a smile, but the effect is the same. Jokes put the audience in a better mood and make them more receptive to what you are saying. Berating the audience actually insults them by implying that they're too dumb to understand the story you just told, and as a consequence, you'll lose them.

• Don't stand and wait for laughter. A long pause waiting for a laugh indicates that you expected it, and because it did not come through, you are unsure of what to do. Most experienced speakers prepare several one-liners to follow up the failure of a joke, one of which may be used in such a case. If you watch comedians, you will recognize a number of common ones—and hackneyed ones—that you probably have heard over and over, such as "There must be people out there; I can hear the breathing" or "I told my wife that wasn't funny but she made me tell it," and I have seen speakers take out a 3″ x 5″ card and tear it up indicating that they were destroying the story forever. But in the absence of a good follow-up line, simply proceed to the next point in your talk without waiting.

Humor is a delightful, entertaining, and appreciated addition to a talk. Just be sure you do it well and do not lose your audience in the process.

Epilogue

My goal in writing this book has been to get you, the reader, from the preface to the epilogue without discouraging you and, hopefully, to give you some helpful hints along the way.

Those of you who had not considered the many facets that make up a professional speech may have been surprised at the multiple, almost disparate, components. The minutiae of speech preparation, the personality of the speaker, the use of voice, and the dynamics of the locale are but a few of the important considerations—all these and more.

I hope you have gleaned some gems from these pages. Try a few of these suggestions, and when they work, come back and help yourself to more. That is the road to successful professional speaking.

To an inquiry from a passing motorist, "How do I get to Carnegie Hall?"—the wise New Yorker replied, after a thoughtful pause, "Practice . . . practice . . . practice."

Practice! You can do it.

References

Evans, M. (1978). The Abuse of Slides. *British Medical Journal*, 1: 905-908.

Green, S. and Sabler, E. (1977, August). Pro Bono Publico—A Century Later. *American Journal of Public Health,* 67(8): 738.

Haakenson, R. *How to Read a Speech.* Philadelphia: Smith, Kline, and French.

Index

Order Your Own Copy of
This Important Book for Your Personal Library!

PROFESSIONALLY SPEAKING
Public Speaking for Health Professionals

_____ in hardbound at $39.95 (ISBN: 0-7890-0600-6)

_____ in softbound at $19.95 (ISBN: 0-7890-0601-4)

COST OF BOOKS_____	☐ **BILL ME LATER:** ($5 service charge will be added) (Bill-me option is good on US/Canada/Mexico orders only; not good to jobbers, wholesalers, or subscription agencies.)
OUTSIDE USA/CANADA/ MEXICO: ADD 20%_____	
POSTAGE & HANDLING_____ (US: $3.00 for first book & $1.25 for each additional book) Outside US: $4.75 for first book & $1.75 for each additional book)	☐ Check here if billing address is different from shipping address and attach purchase order and billing address information.
	Signature_____
SUBTOTAL_____	☐ **PAYMENT ENCLOSED: $**_____
IN CANADA: ADD 7% GST_____	☐ **PLEASE CHARGE TO MY CREDIT CARD.**
STATE TAX_____ (NY, OH & MN residents, please add appropriate local sales tax)	☐ Visa ☐ MasterCard ☐ AmEx ☐ Discover ☐ Diner's Club
FINAL TOTAL_____ (If paying in Canadian funds, convert using the current exchange rate. UNESCO coupons welcome.)	Account #_____ Exp. Date_____ Signature_____

Prices in US dollars and subject to change without notice.

NAME _____

INSTITUTION _____

ADDRESS _____

CITY _____

STATE/ZIP _____

COUNTRY _____ COUNTY (NY residents only) _____

TEL _____ FAX _____

E-MAIL_____
May we use your e-mail address for confirmations and other types of information? ☐ Yes   ☐ No

Order From Your Local Bookstore or Directly From
The Haworth Press, Inc.
10 Alice Street, Binghamton, New York 13904-1580 • USA
TELEPHONE: 1-800-HAWORTH (1-800-429-6784) / Outside US/Canada: (607) 722-5857
FAX: 1-800-895-0582 / Outside US/Canada: (607) 772-6362
E-mail: getinfo@haworthpressinc.com
PLEASE PHOTOCOPY THIS FORM FOR YOUR PERSONAL USE.

BOF96

FORTHCOMING and NEW BOOKS FROM THE HAWORTH PRESS
ADVANCES in PSYCHOLOGY and MENTAL HEALTH

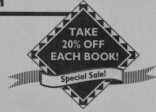

TAKE 20% OFF EACH BOOK!

Special Sale!

INTRODUCTION TO GROUP THERAPY
A Practical Guide

Scott Simon Fehr, PsyD

NEW! Over 250 Pages!

This book combines not only theory and practice, but also practical suggestions in areas that are rarely covered in academic settings in a thorough and well-organized manner.

Contents: Why Group Therapy • The Group Therapist • Group Contract • Self-Protection • Displacement • Dissociation • Emotional Insulation • Identification • Intellectualization • Introjection • Projection • Rationalization • Regression • Repression • Transference and Its Relationship to Group Therapy • Rational Emotive Behavior Therapy • Psychoanalytic Psychotherapy • Basic Assumption Model • Reality Therapy • The Modern Group Analytic Approach • The Problematic Client • Humor and Its Relationship to Psychotherapy • Group Therapy for the Group Therapist • Appendix A • Appendix B • Glossary • Index • Reference Notes Included • *more*

$49.95 hard. ISBN: 0-7890-0612-X.
Text price (5+ copies): $24.95.
Available Spring 1999. Approx. 254 pp. with Index.
Features case studies, diagnostic criteria, chapter review questions, and a glossary.

Make public speaking a cinch by tuning in to the down-to-earth techniques and longtime observations of this well-respected author!

PROFESSIONALLY SPEAKING
Public Speaking for Health Professionals

Arnold Melnick, DO

NEW!

The author covers many important aspects of public speaking, including types of talks, how to prepare your talk, how to deliver your talk, the use of slides, the use of humor, the use of voice, and how to correctly introduce another speaker, among others.

Contents: Preface • Types of Medical Talks • Writing a Medical Speech • Preparing the Manuscript • The Setting • The Speaker • The Talk • Voice and Delivery • Reading a Speech • Use of Audio Visual Aids • Introductions • Being a Program Moderator • Humor in Medical Speaking • Index • Reference Notes Included

$39.95 hard. ISBN: 0-7890-0600-6.
$19.95 soft. ISBN: 0-7890-0601-4.
Available Fall 1998. Approx. 139 pp. with Index.
Features anecdotes, categories and methods of writing and delivering speeches, and figures.

Textbooks are available for classroom adoption consideration on a 60-day examination basis. You will receive an invoice payable within 60 days along with the book. **If you decide to adopt the book, your invoice will be cancelled.** Please write to us on your institutional letterhead, indicating the textbook you would like to examine as well as the following information: course title, current text, enrollment, and decision date.

You can understand the brain's role in identity formation and resultant clinical syndromes to ensure a comprehensive framework for diagnosing and treating your patients!

Over 400 Pages!

HOW THE BRAIN TALKS TO ITSELF
A Clinical Primer of Psychotherapeutic Neuroscience

Jay E. Harris, MD

Synthesizes recent discoveries in cognitive neuroscience with a psychoanalytic understanding of human dynamics and a working model for clinical diagnosis.

Contents: How Do We Evoke and Sense Our Past? • The Stuggle of a Higher Consciousness • The Neural Regulation of Experience • What Happens When Our Identity Is Threatened? • The Roots of Emotional Organization • How Can Therapy Induce Change? • What Is the Near-Death Experience? • What Fosters Addiction? • The Theory of Obsessive-Compulsive Disorder • Where Does the Mind Go When We Lose It? • How the Brain Reveals Its Mental Status • Diagnostic Interviewing • Anorexia and Bulimia • Social Judgment • How to Do Structural Therapy • Notes • Bibliography • Index • *more*

$69.95 hard. ISBN: 0-7890-0408-9.
$39.95 soft. ISBN: 0-7890-0409-7.
1998. Available now. 428 pp. with Index.
Features charts/figures and case studies.

Discover how to cross the boundaries of social differences to deliver effective therapy to your Arab, Asian, and Latin American clients!

CROSS-CULTURAL COUNSELING
The Arab-Palestinian Case

Marwan Adeeb Dwairy, DSc

NEW! Over 200 Pages!

The valuable insight you'll gain into the sociopolitical background and psychocultural features of Arab people and the psychological implications of Arab traditional collectivistic society will help you be more efficient and successful and decrease drop-out rates when treating non-Western clients.

Contents: Mental Health in Arabic Society and Other South/Eastern Cultures • Arab Cultural Attitudes Towards Mental Health • Applying Psychotherapy with South/Eastern Clients • Appendix • References • Index • *more*

$39.95 hard. ISBN: 0-7890-0156-X.
$19.95 soft. ISBN: 0-7890-0481-X.
1998. Available now. 225 pp. with Index.
Features case studies, figures/tables, appendixes, and a bibliography.

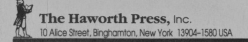

The Haworth Press, Inc.
10 Alice Street, Binghamton, New York 13904-1580 USA

Cure yourself of legal, professional, and ethical phobias concerning your psychotherapy practice!

THE VULNERABLE THERAPIST

Practicing Psychotherapy in an Age of Anxiety

Over 250 Pages!

Helen W. Coale, MSW, LCSW, LMFT

This book will capture your interest with its broad systemic approach, contextual analysis, fascinating case studies, and anecdotal material.

Contents: The Need for Transformation in the Mental Health Professions • Social Constructionism and Its Implications for the Mental Health Professions • Professional Resistance to Feminist Revisions of Diagnosis • Ideas About the Self • Legal Vulnerability Licensing Boards, Malpractice Actions, and Profiles of Complaints • Sudden and Unpredictable Crises and Events • The Character of the Therapist • The Ethical Therapist • References • Index • *more*

$49.95 hard. ISBN: 0-7890-0179-9.
$24.95 soft. ISBN: 0-7890-0480-1.
1998. Available now. 272 pp. with Index.
Features case studies and extensive references.

CALL OUR TOLL-FREE NUMBER: 1–800–HAWORTH
US & Canada only / 8am–5pm ET; Monday–Friday
Outside US/Canada: + 607–722–5857

FAX YOUR ORDER TO US: 1–800–895–0582
Outside US/Canada: + 607–771–0012

E-MAIL YOUR ORDER TO US:
getinfo@haworthpressinc.com

VISIT OUR WEB SITE AT:
http://www.haworthpressinc.com

TAKE 20% OFF EACH BOOK!
Special Sale!

Psychotherapy's search for a high-order theory that explicates its behavioral, biological, and cognitive foundations is over!

BEYOND THE THERAPEUTIC RELATIONSHIP

Behavioral, Biological, and Cognitive Foundations of Psychotherapy

Over 300 Pages!

Frederic J. Leger, MEd
Foreword by Arnold A. Lazarus, PhD

Cuts across multivarious therapies to create an integrated, high-order theory that unites psychotherapy's disparate forces.

Contents: Delineating Psychotherapeutic Variables • The Therapeutic versus Interpersonal Relationship • Facilitative versus Growth-Inhibiting Behaviors • Eye Contact Research in Psychotherapy • Intensive Experiential Exploration • Self-Disclosure as Therapeutic • The Talking Cure • Language as a Bridge Between Mind and Brain • Mind, Brain, and the Generation of Consciousness Through Language • Scientific Roadblocks • Facilitative Nonverbal Interaction in Psychotherapy • Helping Clients "Shoulder the Burden of Change" • Bibliography • Index • *more*

$49.95 hard. ISBN: 0-7890-0291-4.
$24.95 soft. ISBN: 0-7890-0292-2.
1998. 330 pp. with Index. **Includes a bibliography.**

Visit our online catalog and search for publications of interest to you by title, author, keyword, or subject! You'll find descriptions, reviews, and complete tables of contents of books and journals!
http://www.haworthpressinc.com

Order Today and Save!

TITLE	ISBN	REGULAR PRICE	20%-OFF PRICE

• Discount available only in US, Canada, and Mexico and not available in conjunction with any other offer.
• Individual orders outside US, Canada, and Mexico must be prepaid by check, credit card, or money order.
• In Canada: Add 7% for GST after postage & handling.
• Outside USA, Canada, and Mexico: Add 20%.
• MN, NY, and OH residents: Add appropriate local sales tax.

Please complete information below or tape your business card in this area.

NAME _____

ADDRESS _____

_____

CITY _____

STATE _____ ZIP _____

COUNTRY _____

COUNTY (NY residents only) _____

TEL _____ FAX _____

E-MAIL _____
May we use your e-mail address for confirmations and other types of information?
( ) Yes ( ) No. We appreciate receiving your e-mail address and fax number. Haworth would like to e-mail or fax special discount offers to you, as a preferred customer. We will never **share, rent, or exchange** your e-mail address or fax number. We regard such actions as an invasion of your privacy.

POSTAGE AND HANDLING:	
If your book total is:	Add
up to $29.95	$5.00
$30.00 – $49.99	$6.00
$50.00 – $69.99	$7.00
$70.00 – $89.99	$8.00
$90.00 – $109.99	$9.00
$110.00 – $129.99	$10.00
$130.00 – $149.99	$11.00
$150.00 and up	$12.00

• US orders will be shipped via UPS; Outside US orders will be shipped via Book Printed Matter. For shipments via other delivery services, contact Haworth for details. Based on US dollars. Booksellers: Call for freight charges. • If paying in Canadian funds, please use the current exchange rate to convert total to Canadian dollars. • Payment in UNESCO coupons welcome. • Please allow 3-4 weeks for delivery after publication. • Prices and discounts subject to change without notice. • Discount not applicable on books priced under $15.00.

❏ **BILL ME LATER** ($5 service charge will be added).
(Bill-me option available on US/Canadian/Mexican orders only. Not available for subscription agencies. Service charge is waived for booksellers/wholesalers/jobbers.)

Signature _____

❏ PAYMENT ENCLOSED _____
(Payment must be in US or Canadian dollars by check or money order drawn on a US or Canadian bank.)

❏ PLEASE CHARGE TO MY CREDIT CARD:
❏ VISA ❏ MASTERCARD ❏ AMEX ❏ DISCOVER ❏ DINERS CLUB

Account # _____ Exp Date _____

Signature _____
May we open a confidential credit card account for you for possible future purchases? ( ) Yes ( ) No

The Haworth Press, Inc. (24) 08/98 BBC98
10 Alice Street, Binghamton, New York 13904-1580 USA